THE FOCUS EFFECT

the focus effect

CHANGE YOUR WORK, CHANGE YOUR LIFE

Greg Wells Ph.D. & Bruce Bowser

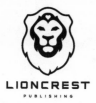

LIONCREST

PUBLISHING

THE FOCUS EFFECT

Change Your Work, Change Your Life

ISBN   978-1-5445-1061-3 *Paperback*

978-1-5445-1060-6 *Ebook*

Contents

Introduction

Think back to the not-so-distant past, before handheld access to all the world's information was in everyone's back pocket.

Imagine sitting down to dinner with your spouse, settling back into your chair, and pulling out a newspaper from which you do not look up for the duration of the meal.

Imagine walking into a business meeting with important clients and asking them to wait for a few moments while you text or email a note to someone else.

Imagine reaching out to a coworker long after most people go to bed with a quick thought or small piece of information that easily could have waited until the next day.

No one in his or her right mind would ever do any of these things, at least not if they wanted to stay married, keep that client, or maintain a civil relationship with that colleague. Yet such behavior is not only commonplace today but is widely acceptable. With the prevalence of smartphones, it is assumed everyone is expected to constantly check their email, even after work hours and even if they are not being paid to do so. Digital media has swept in to define our sense of what is appropriate. We are never out of reach; we are never unplugged. And we are paying for it, both on a personal level and as it pertains to our work performance because we are constantly distracted.

The addiction to distraction and all it entails—including the incessant inundation of text messages, social media, television, and email—has the potential to cause mental health challenges, while also having the potential to be powerfully positive if used the right way. One of the biggest causes of anxiety and distress is the constant overload we face every day. It leads to higher levels of frustration, as perceptions of increased effort required to do fewer tasks leaves us feeling burned out and exhausted.

When we consider the long-term effect of all this distraction, we can't help but wonder what the future will look like for our children. Many parents use iPads and other digital devices to pacify and occupy their young children. These parents are inadvertently creating an atmosphere where children are no longer engaging in conversations or storytelling. They are learning the art of digital communication, which is not a bad thing in and of itself, but it often comes at the expense of learning how to actually converse with another human being. Sherry Turkle, author of *Alone Together: Why We Expect More from Technology and Less from Each Other*, says while we as humans are talking more than ever thanks to email and social media, we are no longer conversing. We're talking *at* each other rather than *with* each other.

Children model their parents. When they see their parents texting while eating or staring at their phones at the park, they understand that that is acceptable behavior. What are we teaching them when every time they seek our attention, we hand them a device? Many children no longer know how to initiate conversation in person because the adults around them are too absorbed in their handheld devices to engage with others around them.

Such behavior is seemingly unavoidable in today's society. A 2015 survey conducted by the Adobe Campaign team of more than four hundred US-based white-collar workers age eighteen and older found most people use email six hours a day. Nine of ten respondents said they check personal email at work and work email from home. According to an Adobe blog post detailing the findings of the survey,[1] "Americans most commonly check their email

---

1   Kristin Naragon, "Subject: Email, We Just Can't Get Enough," *Adobe Blog*, August 26, 2015, https://blogs.adobe.com/conversations/2015/08/email.html.

while watching TV (70%), from bed (52%), on vacation (50%), while on the phone (43%), from the bathroom (42%) and even—most dangerously—while driving (18%). As for those coveted millennials? They've doubled down on email, both at work and at home. We found that millennials are more mobile and more frequent users of email than any other age group:

- Millennials are more likely to check work email outside of normal work hours.
- One-third are comfortable using emojis to communicate with a direct manager or senior executive.
- Eighty-eight percent use a smartphone to check email.
- Millennials are also more likely than any other age group to check email from bed (70%), from the bathroom (57%) or while driving (27%)."

THE CULT OF BUSYNESS

When we let such distractions dictate how we live our lives, we are giving in to what we call the Cult of Busyness. We believe we always have to be reachable, always have to be multitasking, always have to be on. The ironic result of living like this is that we end up more distracted than ever. (More on the Cult of Busyness in chapter 5.)

The simple act of sitting down to focus on one task is becoming increasingly difficult for most people. Distraction is destroying our ability to do our best work on the things that matter most to us, whether it's career, school, business, or avocation. Many people today are so used to communicating in 144 characters or fewer that it is hard for them to focus on more than that. We'll never be able to achieve to the best of our abilities unless we learn how to focus.

The average person spends more than sixty hours a year just looking to see if they have a text or email, not actually reading it. Imagine what you could do with an extra sixty hours a year or ninety minutes each week. You could work out, go for a walk, meditate, or just be with family. You could do anything you wanted. When you make time for the things that really matter, you begin to leave the Cult of Busyness behind and take steps toward a more fulfilling life.

DRIVEN TO DISTRACTION

We are living through a cultural change similar to what happened during the Industrial Revolution one hundred years ago. The advent of machinery required the creation of factories, and the majority of the population shifted its focus from agriculture to industry. Today, there are more mobile phones in the world than there are toilets. A relatively small percentage of the population of India has access to water and power, yet the majority of the population now has a cell phone.

We are in the early days of the internet revolution. We are ten years into something that will drastically change the way we live and work for the next one hundred years, if not longer. As a result, we are seeing a massive cultural shift, but it is nothing compared to what is coming. Artificial intelligence is going to disrupt everything from the way we drive to how medicine and law are practiced.

According to an October 2016 *Harvard Business Review* article, "Technology Will Replace Many Doctors, Lawyers, and Other Professionals," there are now "more monthly visits to the WebMD network, a collection of health websites, than to all the doctors in the United States. Annually, in the world of disputes, 60 million disagreements among eBay traders are resolved using 'online dispute resolution' rather than lawyers and judges—this is three times the number of lawsuits filed each year in the entire U.S. court system. The U.S. tax authorities in 2014 received electronic tax returns from almost 50 million people who had relied on online tax-preparation software rather than human tax professionals."[2]

The topic of the Cult of Busyness is on the mind of every corporate leader, human resources officer, and business owner. Studies show average North Americans spend

---

2   Richard Susskind and Daniel Susskind, "Technology Will Replace Many Doctors, Lawyers, and Other Professionals," *Harvard Business Review*, October 11, 2016, https://hbr.org/2016/10/robots-will-replace-doctors-lawyers-and-other-professionals.

30–40 percent of their day distracted, which is costing the United States $900 billion a year. The average person spends nearly two hours on social media every day.[3]

A 2014 Virgin Pulse report titled *Driven by Distraction: Why Employees' Focus Is Waning at Work and What You Can Do about It*, shows that of the employees surveyed, 43 percent said they were distracted for 21–75 percent or more of their workday. Of those distracted employees, 45 percent said tech disruptions, such as email and text messages, were the top distracters, and 31 percent said online activities not related to work, including shopping, social media, and reading blogs, hampered their productivity.[4]

Distraction has long been a problem, well before the advent of the smartphone. People have always found ways to focus on something other than the task at hand. Digital technology is, in the scope of human history, very new. The iPhone is only ten years old. But in those ten years, technology and social media have crept in to affect nearly everything we do. A decade ago, no one filmed a concert. The audience just enjoyed it. Now, in this age

3   Evan Asano, "How Much Time Do People Spend on Social Media?" *Social Media Today*, January 4, 2017, https://www.socialmediatoday.com/marketing/how-much-time-do-people-spend-social-media-infographic.

4   Alyssa Azevedo, "Wonder Why Employees' Focus Keep Waning?" *Virgin Pulse*, October 22, 2014, https://www.virginpulse.com/blog-post/wonder-employees-focus-keeps-waning-infographic/.

of "pics or it didn't happen," everyone films the event to share it on social media.

We need to learn how to navigate this new landscape, where we have the entire history of the world's knowledge in our pocket. This shift is having an impact on all of humanity, but if we learn how to best navigate the change, we can take advantage of it instead of being a slave to it.

We believe technology is an amazing tool for humankind and that, in many ways, it holds the keys to our survival as a species. We need to use technology to our advantage. We want to see people talking again, engaging with each other over a meal, not walking around like zombies glued to their devices. We want everyone to be able to disconnect long enough to reclaim their evenings, weekends, and family time. We want people to be able to use their mobile devices to change the world for the better, without experiencing any negative health effects.

HOW DID WE GET HERE?

Unfortunately, in today's world, disengaging from distraction is not so simple. The ubiquitous nature of smartphones means a world of distraction is always within reach. Most children today take in more information in one week than their great-great-grandparents did in their entire lifetimes. Two or three generations ago, people would have to obtain and read a newspaper, or gather in a public meeting to share information. Today, we are inundated with breaking news.

Whether it's checking news, engaging in social media, or texting, most of us are guilty of excessive checking, even when it's not entirely appropriate. Just look at how we lived a few short years ago versus how we live today. People walk around in public looking at their phones all the time. How many times have you had to dodge a person who was walking and texting, oblivious to the world around them? Every so often, I'll let somebody get close to me just to see their reaction. Almost always, they give me a look of scorn as if they're thinking, *Hey, can't you see I'm texting and walking? Get out of my way!*

Distraction is an epidemic affecting all of humankind, including us (the authors). We've both had moments when we realized a lack of focus was affecting how we were living our lives.

GREG'S STORY

As a professor, scientist, author, public speaker, and owner of a consulting company, I usually have a rather busy schedule. I also have a young family and do my best to spend high-quality time with them.

Several years ago, I was at the park with my daughter, who was four at the time. As she was playing, I was checking my email. She came over to me and used a line from her favorite movie, *Shrek*, to call out my bad behavior. "Daddy," she said, "your job is not my problem," quoting Princess Fiona when she's just about had it with her ogre companion.

It was a shocking moment for me. There was my daughter, telling me she'd like to have some of my attention when I had my nose buried in my phone. I was devastated. I put the phone away.

Ever since that day, I've been deliberate about my actions. Now, when I play with my kids, not only am I there physically, but I am also there mentally. I am present. Conversely, when I have to work, I tell them, "Daddy actually has to go do work now. I'll be back in an hour. Don't interrupt me. I'm going to my office. My office is off-limits. If you need anything urgently, come knock on the door."

They now know the boundaries. When I'm with them, I'm with them. When I'm working, I'm working. My personal life and my work life are no longer all meshed together.

While it took that moment with my daughter for me to understand how focus can improve my own life, I'd witnessed its power for many years in my profession. As a physiologist, I have had the opportunity to work with hundreds of Olympians during the course of twenty years. In 2010 and 2012, I was asked to be the sports science and sports medicine analyst for Canadian television during the Olympic Games in Vancouver and London. My role in the segments was to analyze the difference between the medalists and their less-successful competitors.

From a physical standpoint, most Olympic athletes are in a reasonably level playing field, with the exception of a few notables, such as Michael Phelps and Usain Bolt.

In my observation, the one factor determining whether athletes are going to be successful in their event is their focus—their ability to control their attention. The potential for distraction at the Olympics is relentless. Someone is always asking for your time. You have to manage the media, your sponsors, your family, your teammates, your coaches, and the crowd.

The athletes who are able to say no to unnecessary demands and put their full focus on achieving their goals go on to win. You can instantly tell whether athletes are going to do well at the Olympics based on their social media feeds. If they are able to resist posting, turn off their devices, and just focus on performance, they have a much greater chance at success. Based on these observations, I contributed to several powerful segments on how athletes use focus to prepare and perform.

I also like to study how humans perform in various extreme circumstances. As part of my research, I embark on an expedition every few years. In 2016, I climbed Chimborazo, a volcano in Ecuador. At about twenty-one thousand feet, a mile higher than Everest, Chimborazo is the farthest point from Earth's center.

During one of our practice runs, we had reached about 18,500 feet when the temperature dropped drastically. The winds shifted. I began to experience the symptoms of altitude sickness. My head began to pound and my vision blurred. I had to descend the volcano with minimal vision. It was brutal. It became a life-or-death situation. I knew getting down was going to take every bit of focus I had. If I lost it even for a moment, I could die. With a five thousand-foot drop on either side of me, I put my eyes on the boots of the person in front of me, and focused on nothing else for the next few hours until we reached the bottom.

As we descended and the oxygen levels went back up again, I gradually regained my eyesight, and the headache went away. As I began to feel better, I realized the scenario was an analogy for what you must do anytime you're under pressure. You have to focus on the single most important thing and not worry about anything else.

BRUCE'S STORY

As the father of two grown daughters, I have a vested interest in changing the way society reconciles its addiction to distraction. The unnecessary stress and anxiety my daughters and the rest of their generation will experience because of the digital age they live in is of great concern to me, and I've witnessed its effects firsthand.

On a regular basis, my daughters and I meet for a father-daughter dinner and have for years. For these dinners, we always try to find a nice restaurant with a great wine list. At our dinners, I noticed we would all be there, drinking our wine and enjoying a good meal, every single one of us texting and checking messages the entire time.

Last year, I suggested to my daughters, "If we're going to have a really nice dinner, can we agree to give our phones to the server until we're finished with dinner?"

"Seriously?" they replied.

After some prodding, we all agreed to turn our phones on silent and give them to the server for the duration of the meal. It changed our dinners. We began to engage and have complete conversations rather than squeezing in talking between texts. We noticed time went by quickly, we smiled more, and we left feeling relaxed and reconnected. Isn't that what having dinner with loved ones is supposed to be like? Sadly, many of us have lost the art of conversation, and there is no time like now to get it back.

I also realized I could benefit from improved focus when I went back to school a few years ago to complete a degree I'd started more than thirty years before. I found it was incredibly difficult for me to sit still long enough to read the required materials, because I was so used to being distracted. Every time a notification popped up on my computer, I checked it. Every time a text came through, I read it. I was getting nowhere.

I decided to take action. When I needed to study on campus, I told my family I would be unreachable for those hours unless they called the library. My daughters have become accustomed to reaching me on demand, which is not their fault as I have created that expectation, so I had to explain I was going offline for a couple of hours, and if it was an emergency, they could call the university. The good news for most of us is that emergencies are few and far between.

I started setting specific hours for checking email and did not open it outside the designated time frame. I had to stop being constantly connected or I wasn't going to be able to function.

It made a huge difference. My anxiety level dropped. My

attention span increased significantly. I became far more productive. When I was disconnected and focusing on a specific task, such as writing a paper, I got into a zone or flow where time went by quickly. The papers were better, and I felt better. I was being present and focused.

I've experienced a similar level of focused attention when pursuing my hobby of flying airplanes. When you are flying, you must be totally focused on what you're doing or things can go bad very quickly. Because of the attention it demands, flying becomes almost meditative for me. I go up, and time stands still. I come back feeling more relaxed and less anxious. You can't look at your phone or check your emails when flying an airplane. Again, I am being present and focused. You need to be totally focused, which is exactly what we're missing in the workplace today. People are not focused on a single task long enough to make true progress.

I've been the CEO of AMJ Campbell Van Lines for nearly twenty-five years. We're in an older industry, but I've always tried to incorporate cutting-edge practices into the way we do things, whether engaging employees or delivering service. For me, addressing the issue of distraction in the workplace is less about squeezing more productivity out of people, and more about creating a world where employees are healthier, less distracted, and leading happier lives. It's not about turning a better profit or expecting employees to act like robots, operating at an unreasonably high level. It's about making the workplace better for both employer and employee, and allowing everyone to enjoy the benefits of a place where extreme importance is placed on everyone's overall well-being.

THE FOCUS EFFECT

Companies must begin to develop cultures where distraction is no longer draining energy and stealing productivity. Several months ago, we began researching and implementing practices to help get ourselves and our teams focused to work smarter, not harder.

Our dream and vision are to provide you with the information, tools, tactics, and strategies you need to change your work and your life for the better. At work, we want you to increase your performance, enjoy more success, have more energy, and be healthier both mentally and physically. We would love for you to use stress to your advantage, be happier and to have less anxiety and more excitement. Ideally, we would all have fewer distractions and more focus on a daily basis. We want you to be present—both at work and with your family—because that is the key to a world-class life. We want you to crush it at work and then be able to take real vacations so you can experience all the world has to offer while recovering and regenerating. Companies whose employees use these strategies will be more profitable, will perform at a higher level more consistently, and will navigate the ups and downs of markets better. Companies that embed these principles in their cultures will have better employee engagement and retention, better overall mental health, and ultimately, more success.

We will delve deeper into each facet of what we call the Focus Effect in the coming chapters. We will also have a number of sections in the book we call "Words of Wisdom" from world-class performers who provide their insights into how they applied the Focus Effect in their lives to great effect. Here's a great one from Olympic champion Catriona Le May Doan to get us started:

WORDS OF WISDOM: CATRIONA LE MAY DOAN

Catriona Le May Doan is an Olympic champion speed skater from Canada who is generally considered to be one of the greatest in history. For her, focus is a must that comes very naturally.

"If I didn't focus on achieving the ultimate performance in training, then I'd be disappointed in myself," she says. "I had my goal, and I was a perfectionist, so that was the focus in training."

Le May Doan even showed focus when resting, although in a more outward manner. When she was resting, she focused on music and her relationships. She perceived those as her reward after and between intervals. When she was competing, that focus turned inward. Her races were thirty-seven seconds long—no time could be wasted on a wandering mind.

"In racing, I really had to train myself," she says. "I had to learn that when you're having a good race, everything that happens on the ice just happens, and awareness was there, and that I was OK."

To get into that deep bubble of focus in competitions and avoid becoming distracted by the crowd and the TV crews, Le May Doan had five technical words she wrote on a piece of paper. She would reread them right before she went out to race to remind herself of the only thing that mattered. She then tried to enjoy the moment and listen for her teammates cheering. The best races, she remembers, happened when she was relaxed.

"Every time the focus shifted to a competitor, I had a bad race, and the race was over," she says. "When we focus on others, we lose the ability to perform and reach our potential because we start judging. For me, it was all about learning how to excel leading into a race. I could literally see that piece of paper with the race written out in five words. If I focused only on that, then I could get into the flow and enjoy it."

HOW WE CAN HELP YOU

This book will help you construct world-class routines and habits by building a high-performance, healthy, and happy life both at home and at work. It will delve into the physical and psychological impact of distraction and offer tools based on our own firsthand experiences and research to help you reshape the way you and your organization approach the workday.

Our goal is to help employees become superstars and help employers create high-performance workplaces where people want to work, not *have* to work. Some of the fastest-growing companies are attracting and retaining top talent by providing employees with work-life balance opportunities and creating environments where employees are given all the tools to be their best, everything from healthy food options to shorter and more flexible work hours and days. They are breaking the mold of the old way of doing things and succeeding because of it.

Employers can use the practices detailed in this book to change any industry and create environments that allow them to compete for the young and bright talent. Employees can use this book to up their performance by changing the way they work, avoiding unnecessary distraction, eating better, working smarter, and staying on task.

We are writing for entrepreneurs, business leaders,

employees, and individuals who want to be a step ahead of the game. This is not meant to be just another book on the shelf but rather the beginning of a movement that addresses the global distraction crisis in a meaningful way. We want to start moving the pendulum back to create better parents, happier spouses, and healthier employees. This is not a ripple but a wave that will help people all over the world unlock their potential.

As coauthors, we will each share personal stories while maintaining a first-person point of view. Our shared experience will help you learn how to minimize distraction and improve focus so you can compete favorably in the global marketplace with the Googles and Zapposes of the world.

GREG AND BRUCE'S 1% TIPS

As you work through all the information, advice, and suggestions in this book, keep focused on micro-improvements. A 1% change may not seem like much, but each one takes you, step by step, further along the path to your best life. Throughout the book, you will find a series of 1% Tips. Practice them and share them with your family, friends, and community.

PART 1

Personal Mastery

. . . .

Most people live within the confines of their comfort zone. The best thing you can do for yourself is to regularly move beyond it. This is the way to lasting personal mastery and to realize the true potential of your human endowments.

—ROBIN SHARMA

CHAPTER 1

From Distraction to Focus

Digital technology has evolved at a breakneck pace since the emergence of the smartphone a decade ago. Hundreds of apps have been developed since, each vying for our attention. People spend significant parts of their days checking social media. They provide a way for everyone to be constantly engaged but distracted at the same time, even though the information they provide is usually mindless. Just look at how popular posts about food are. If I post a picture of my dinner, it gets more interaction than anything else I do.

The addiction to social media does make sense from a physiological perspective. You get a dopamine hit every time you check social media and see that somebody liked your post. You also hear stories about young people who become depressed because they're not getting many likes on their posts. Social media can be very useful and beneficial, but not when it begins to control you. Unfortunately, more and more of us are letting that happen.

Email can be just as harmful when you allow it to constantly rob you of your focus. I was once doing a consulting session with a CEO of a large organization. We were discussing strategies for decreasing stress. During our conversation, his computer would ping every thirty seconds or so. I watched him twitch each time.

I asked him to pause. I reached over, turned off the sound on his computer, and shut down the monitor. He was taken aback. I said, "Don't worry about it. It's just for a few minutes." Within two to three minutes, his entire physiology changed. His shoulders dropped. He actually looked at me. We connected. He could have a deep conversation, and as a result, we were able to solve many of his problems.

Had I not done that, his mind would have been constantly shifting back to his work. Something as simple as turning off a notification can be a powerful tool for improving your life.

WHAT HAPPENS WHEN WE'RE DISTRACTED

Imagine you are sitting on a bench engrossed in a book. I

sit down beside you and interrupt you. We chat for a few minutes. When I leave, do you go back to the exact line where you left off? Not likely. You'll go back two, three, or four paragraphs to reorient yourself and remind your brain where you are.

The same thing happens when you are on task and become distracted. Recent research shows it can take a minimum of four to eight minutes to get back into whatever you were doing.

Anytime you are engaged in an activity, the brain becomes activated and neurons begin to fire. They create electricity, which moves through them and triggers the release of chemicals. This brain activation requires a great deal of energy. Although the brain makes up only 2 percent of the body's weight, it uses 20 percent of the body's energy.

We deliver that energy through blood flow, which gives us the oxygen and glucose the brain uses to concentrate, problem solve, and be creative. When we are doing a task, certain parts of the brain and specific neurons are activated. Blood flow goes to that location to supply it with oxygen and nutrients so it can work.

If we task-switch and jump back and forth between activities, different parts of the brain are activated. As a result, blood flow has to move from one location to another, and that takes time. You activate one part of the brain and deliver nutrients to it, and then you shut that part down and open up another. Therefore, multitasking is actually a highly inefficient process for the brain. It simply doesn't work that way.

> ### 1% TIP: AVOID RESTARTING A TASK
>
> It takes a significant amount of energy to activate the areas of your brain that are required to perform a task. If you constantly switch from one task to another, just as the blood flow, oxygen, and glucose for the current task are arriving, you are activating another part of your brain. And when you return to the original task, you will have to go through the activation process once more. This is highly inefficient. As much as possible, stay with a task you start by avoiding distractions while working.

It also constantly shifts us into sympathetic activations. We have two nervous systems inside our body: the sympathetic system, which is our fight-or-flight response and important for doing physical and mental work; and the parasympathetic system, our recovery and regeneration system.

According to the 2009 *Harvard Business Review* article, "Death by Information Overload," the inundation of available information can actually lower people's intelligence. The article cites a study commissioned by Hewlett-Packard that shows IQ scores of knowledge workers distracted by email and phone calls fell an average of ten points.[5]

Every time you check your phone or open social media or read an email, you're activating the sympathetic nervous system. When we do it all day long, we are constantly in a state of fight or flight, which can have can serious negative health consequences including burnout, stress, anxiety, and lack of creativity.

This can lead to a great deal of wasted time in the workplace, which is one reason an overhaul of antiquated practices is necessary.

---

5   Paul Hemp, "Death by Information Overload," *Harvard Business Review*, September 2009, https://hbr.org/2009/09/death-by-information-overload.

WORDS OF WISDOM: DR. ISAIAH HANKEL, AUTHOR OF BLACK HOLE FOCUS

Dr. Isaiah Hankel, author of *Black Hole Focus*, spoke with Greg about taking back your time. An excerpt from the discussion follows:

You need to fight for some of your own time. People come up with all kinds of excuses for why they can't set aside fifteen minutes to themselves, but if you look at the research, it's very clear: the only way to really be successful in life is to continue to create better and better habits for yourself, free up more of your time and be more productive.

Studies also show that in terms of productive time during the day, you have only about 90 minutes to 120 minutes maximum productive time. It does not matter who you are. The question is, what are you doing with this time?

Are you protecting those hours? A good way to get started is by creating a new habit. It doesn't have to be big. If you try to start by going to the gym every day and doing thirty sets of exercises, that's too much. You'll get bogged down by all the new small habits that are a part of that one big habit you're trying to do. It makes it hard to follow and turn into an automatic process.

Instead, start with a tiny habit. Go to the gym and do one set of one exercise. Do that for a week, and then add two sets or three sets. After a few weeks, add five or six sets.

The key is to know when your peak mental energy is and create a habit for utilizing it. Start with fifteen minutes. If you're at your best in the morning, get up fifteen minutes earlier by yourself. Map out what you want during that time. If you do that for seven days in row, you're almost at two hours of complete focus time. The results can be absolutely dramatic.

CHAPTER 2

Master Your Morning

There are several ways we can invite focus into our daily lives while also driving away distractions. Having a plan and executing it until it becomes routine allows us to set ourselves up for success each and every day.

Approach your day with the same careful planning and consideration a pilot must exercise when preparing for a flight. You don't only start thinking about the journey ahead when you're barreling down the runway. You must have a preflight checklist to make sure all the elements are in place for a successful flight.

A morning routine can act as your own preflight checklist. By doing each item on the list, you are setting yourself up to be at your best for the day ahead.

WIN THE MORNING, WIN THE DAY

A consistent morning routine is critical. If we look at all the elite performers in the world regardless of discipline, many are early risers who rely on routines to ensure they are controlling as many variables as possible. They do the same things every day and adjust their routines depending on outcomes, which enables them to be constantly improving.

If a morning routine is a new concept for you, start by making yourself a checklist including the following activities in whatever order works best for you: morning affirmation, meditation, fuel, and exercise. Doing all these things takes only about an hour if you are diligent, and if you wake up early enough, you can easily get them all done by 7:00 a.m. (and if you still think you don't have enough time for them, read over the No Excuses section in chapter 4).

1% TIP: FOLLOW A PRODUCTIVE MORNING ROUTINE

Commit to a morning routine that will set you up for success and then write it down in a checklist to follow. You can then begin each day by going through these activities and ensure you are energized and focused on what you want to accomplish. In particular, consider a morning routine that includes all of the following: an affirmation, a brief meditation, nutritious and energizing fuel, and stimulating exercise.

MORNING AFFIRMATION

A morning affirmation is something you can do as soon as you wake up. It takes only seconds but can set the tone for the rest of your day.

Take a moment to establish your intentions for the day and form a positive statement. It can be something as simple as, "This is going to be a great day," or "I'm super happy to be alive." You might tell yourself, "I'm going to change the world today," or "Today is another chance to achieve all my goals."

These might sound cheesy, but thinking intentionally about these kinds of statements first thing in the morning can set your mindset and establish control over your day from the get-go.

MINDFULNESS AND MEDITATION

While the words *mindfulness* and *meditation* might have once seemed to apply to only a select group of extreme health-minded people, they are now used commonly in business settings as employers realize their significant impact on stress levels, focus, and overall well-being. In recent years, there has been an explosion of resources, from in-person classes to smartphone apps, aimed at helping people center themselves and quiet their minds so they can be more present and more focused.

There are simple ways you can introduce meditation into your daily routine. Download an app, such as Muse, that guides you through quick sessions you can do right at your desk. There are many other apps out there, but we recommend Muse as we have personally met with the founders and find their approach to be highly beneficial.

If you don't have access to an app, simply take a few minutes and simply focus on your breathing. Inhale and exhale, concentrating on each breath. By centering your mind and allowing it to relax and regenerate, just as you would your body, you are giving it the boost it needs to take on the rest of the day.

The health benefits—both mental and physical—of meditation have been proven again and again. It is a great proactive way to combat stress, as you are anticipating the challenges of the coming day and giving your mind the time and space it needs to best prepare to meet them.

If this is a new practice for you, start small. Try it for just a few minutes and work your way up as you feel your ability to focus growing stronger.

If meditation is not for you, try something simple such as a five-minute journaling exercise. Start your day by writing out several things you are grateful for, a few things you are looking forward to, or even just an affirmation. This will also help you clear your mind and put you in a positive mindset for the day ahead.

1% TIP: BEGIN THE DAY MINDFULLY

Start your day with a meditation, mindfulness, or brief journaling session that will focus your mind on the joys of your life and what you are grateful for and help you clear your mind of worry and negative thoughts. Through breathing, relaxation, and affirmations, you can create a clear mind and positive attitude toward the coming day.

FUEL IS THE FOUNDATION

We know nutrition is the foundation for elite mental and physical performance. If you're eating properly, your risk of cancer, heart disease, diabetes, metabolic syndrome, depression, and anxiety decrease dramatically.

Every food and drink choice you make impacts your health. A simple way to start treating your body better is by removing sugars. Every morning, I see lines out the door of my local coffee shop, where people start their days by loading up on scones, pastries, cakes, cookies, and of course, caffeine. Filling your body with so much sugar might give you a temporary jolt, but enjoy it while it lasts. By the time mid-morning rolls around, that burst of energy will be long gone and instead replaced with a feeling of lethargy and dissatisfaction. If you instead opt to start your day with food packed with protein, you not only get something that tastes good, but you also enhance your performance and extend your life.

Also, pay attention to when you eat. Creating a routine helps you avoid eating randomly, which often means snacking or grazing on things you don't really want or need. Don't forage; plan your meals. Know what you will eat when to stay deliberate in all your nutrition choices.

Our bodies need fuel first thing in the morning, and using this as an opportunity to choose something healthy is a great way to start the day with intention. Stick to foods high in protein and fiber, full of healthy fats and complex carbohydrates. Ideal options for the first fuel of the day include lemon ginger tea and green smoothies.

1% TIP: PLAN TO FUEL YOUR BODY FIRST THING

All of us benefit from having a plan for what we eat to avoid snacking, grazing, or making less-than-healthy choices. In particular, try to be deliberate about what you eat in the morning when your body needs fuel to get going. Avoid sugar or simple carbohydrates that will offer a temporary jolt but leave you listless by mid-morning.

It is also important to remember to hydrate. Throughout the night, our bodies lose water simply through breathing. We need to replenish that supply early in the day.

Beginning the day with a heavy meal laden with unhealthy fats and unnecessary calories only weighs us down, literally and figuratively. Don't let your first choice of the day derail you. Give yourself the energy you need to attack the day.

INCREASE ACTIVITY, INCREASE PRODUCTIVITY

Starting the day with a workout is an ideal way to get your brain waves and blood flowing. Cardio activates the brain. Exercising in the morning floods your brain with brain-derived neurotrophic factor (BDNF), which stimulates the growth of new neurons to facilitate learning and memory. Exercise also activates the part of your brain associated with creativity and problem solving. It makes us sharper and more capable of concentration.

There are many ways you can incorporate physical activity into your day; a daily trip to the gym is great for many people, but even a quick walk outside or some stretching as soon as you get out of bed can make a big difference. We are not at our best when we feel weighed down. Exercise, even light movements, gets blood flowing and allows our brains to work faster and better.

Movement improves mental function and also addresses any issues you might have with anxiety or depression. When you consider all the benefits, there is no excuse for avoiding exercise. If it helps, add some accountability by finding a partner or group to walk with each morning. It's always easier to stick to your workout plans if someone else is relying on your participation.

A regular exercise routine will give you more energy as you begin to feel healthier and more active. Physical health feeds mental health and increases your ability to focus. Do whatever is necessary to ensure your health is optimal to start the day.

If necessary, plan workouts into your day. Put them on your calendar. This way, you'll be less likely to skip or forget them. This is particularly important if you travel. It's easy to use a new location or time change to avoid exercise. Remember the benefits, and make it a regular priority. Exercise is one of the most-researched topics with some of the strongest evidence of efficacy, yet it is seldom embraced by business leaders as an important element of employee well-being and productivity.

1% TIP: GET MOVING

Physical activity is strongly correlated with mental functioning and positive mood. Starting your day with some exercise is an ideal way to get your blood and brain moving, ensuring you arrive for work sharp and focused. Also, have a plan for when you will fit in your workouts or just take a walk so that it happens, especially during busy periods.

AVOID EMAIL

Tempting as it may be, do not check your email throughout your morning routine. A high percentage of the population checks their phone first thing in the morning before doing anything else. This is a surefire way to pull focus away from your morning routine, and possibly even guarantee you won't do any of it. You might see a message and think, *I'll just respond to this one*, then you answer another and another, and before you know it, two hours are gone.

As soon as you check your email, you are on someone else's agenda. You instantly go into reaction mode. To construct a different, better life for yourself, you have to break the cycle of what you typically do. Instead of immediately reaching for the phone, take care of yourself first.

Email will steal your time and attention every time you let it. Do not give it the power to prevent you from starting the day in the best way possible.

A NOTE TO NIGHT OWLS

If you are reading this and thinking, *There is no way this will work for me. I am not a morning person*, do not fret. For some people, winning the afternoon or evening is critical. You can still do all these things; just cater them to your own lifestyle.

It does not matter when you start your routine. What's

important is that you start it at the same part of every day. You just need to have an established time when you go into lockdown. If you exercise in the afternoon or evening, use the energy gained to concentrate later in the day. If you are most productive after traditional work hours, leverage that as much as possible.

CHAPTER 3

Master Your Day: Power Work

Another way to create the optimal workday is to do the bulk (if not all) of your work during the hours of the day when you are at your best. This is different for everyone. Some people like to dive in right after their morning routine and bang out several productive hours of work before lunch. Others like to ease into their days and really dig in later in the afternoon. Some people are night owls.

Once you figure out what works for you, control that time. It is a time each day you will invest in your life's most important work. It is your "Power Work" time.

During this time, you will not engage in anything that is not mission critical. You will turn off your phone and close all irrelevant windows on your computer. You will completely block out anything and everything that could possibly take your attention away from the task at hand. You will not do anything administrative, clerical, or non-pressing. Such activities require less mental investment and should be saved for hours outside of Power Work.

During Power Work, we suggest working in sixty- to ninety-minute blocks followed by ten- to thirty-minute breaks. These breaks can consist of meditation, music, games, light reading, or anything else that helps your brain relax and recharge. A critical element of the program we've implemented at our company is opportunities for employees to take "healthy breaks." We encourage them to take the time to go on a mind-clearing walk, or visit a break room where there is little to no activity or noise. We don't encourage them to spend the entire break on their phone. Rather, the time should be spent letting the mind rest and helping the body break out of the seated position.

If you're not sure what will work for you, analyze your patterns. Take a day, break it out by hour, and think about when you typically feel at your best. For me, it's always the morning. I'm fantastic from 7:00 a.m. through 11:00 a.m. Some days, I can stretch it until 1:00 p.m. From 2:00 p.m. to 4:00 p.m., I don't have great energy. Knowing this, I do all my reading, writing, thinking, strategizing, and editing in the morning. I do phone calls, sales meetings, and other things that don't require a deep level of thinking in the afternoon.

This is just me. If you know you're most productive from 7:00 p.m. to 1:00 a.m., make sure you protect that time for that work. Power Work is very individualized. By identifying the times of day when you feel best, you can get much more done in much less time, and you're going to have the highest level of energy for the things most important to you.

1% TIP: BLOCK TIME TO POWER WORK

Determine the time of day that you are most productive and protect this time for uninterrupted focus on your most important tasks. During this time, do not engage in anything that is not mission critical by turning off all notifications and putting systems in place to ensure you are not interrupted. You can then attend to the nonessential tasks during periods of the day when you are likely to have less energy and focus.

SET YOUR INTENTIONS

If you see someone walking along the street talking to themselves without a mobile phone, you might think that person is crazy. I'm going to ask you to add a little crazy to your life. I want you to talk to yourself.

When you wake up in the morning, I want the first thoughts that enter your mind to be positive. Self-talk is a core mental skill that I ensure all my athletes and corporate clients use as often as possible. It's incredibly powerful. Imagine standing in the blocks right before the final of the 100-meter dash in the Olympic stadium. There are eighty thousand people in the stadium watching you and several billion are checking you out on TV. What would you be saying to yourself? Olympic runners will be saying things like, "OK, let's GO!" or "Fast, fast, fast!" or "You've done the training, now it's time to RACE." You won't have many athletes in the blocks saying, "I'm tired," or "Man I have a lot to do today," or "Wow, I feel old." What you think is what you are. You can have only one thought in your head at any given time; make it a positive one, and make sure you start your day that way.

Positive self-talk can change the way your brain and body work for the better. It's the same philosophy behind why parents like to tell their children they are bright and capable of anything—you become what you're told. By talking to yourself in a positive way, you can change the way you think about yourself. Research from Carnegie Mellon University has even shown that self-affirmations help protect against the damaging effects of stress and can improve academic performance and problem-solving ability in underperforming students.[6]

6   J. David Creswell, Janine M. Dutcher, William M. P. Klein, Peter R. Harris, and John M. Levine, "Self-Affirmation Improves Problem-Solving under Stress," *PLOS ONE* 8, no. 5 (2013): e62593.

It feels great when someone compliments you for a job well done, right? You can make yourself feel great, too, just by speaking to yourself nicely about motivating things. Try statements that start with "I can," "I will," or "I am."

When you wake up in the morning, do yourself a favor. Smile and talk to yourself for a minute about how great you are and how you're going to head out into the world and impose your will to make it a better place. Remember, you are what you think.

1% TIP: GIVE YOURSELF A PEP TALK

Positive self-talk can have a significant positive effect on attitude and performance. At the start of your day, before a challenging meeting or presentation, or when the going gets tough, take a moment to remind yourself that you are capable. This will ensure that how you think about yourself is shaped by you, not by what happens around you.

POWER FUEL

During Power Work, you will need Power Fuel to sustain your energy and focus. Just as you started your day with a healthy meal to propel you in the right direction, you need healthy snacks and lunch options to keep you moving forward.

One of the easiest things people can do to perform better, be healthier, and improve their mental performance is to understand how the foods we eat change the way our brains work. The foods you eat during the day change the chemicals the brain uses to communicate with itself. Those chemicals, called neurotransmitters, are made of various types of things from the foods we eat. If we eat foods higher in protein than carbohydrates, we increase the number of neurotransmitters that help us concentrate and stay focused. If we eat foods higher in carbohydrates than protein, we increase the neurotransmitters that widen our focus and help us to relax.

Just think about how you feel an hour after having a kale salad with chicken versus an hour after having a huge plate of pasta. With the salad, you feel much more able to focus and concentrate and have reasonably good energy. If you have the pasta, you probably need a nap.

The food we eat during the workday has an enormous impact on our productivity. We've all been to lunch with that coworker who has a cheeseburger, french fries, and a glass of wine, then goes back to work. How much quality work can he really accomplish? Yet we live in a society obsessed with food—just look at social media to see our fascination with it. For many of us, photos of food are the most-liked posts in our time lines.

There is no doubt the most distracting foods are also the most prevalent, but if we think about the choices we make and do things differently, we can be healthier and dramatically improve our ability to concentrate and stay focused.

Caffeine can help in some cases, but its peak benefits occur thirty to sixty minutes after you ingest it. Its effect lasts for about three hours, but afterward, the withdrawal can have a negative impact on your performance. Because of this, it's important to schedule your caffeine and think about how it will impact your Power Work.

Nutrient-dense foods optimal for Power Fuel include:

- organic grass-fed meats
- cold-water fish
- black beans
- berries
- avocado
- raw nuts
- seeds
- eggs, particularly omelets with greens
- coconut
- kale
- ginger
- carrots

A good example of how you can add Power Fuel into your day is to eat a little bit of dark chocolate in the afternoon. Chocolate with 70 percent or more cocoa can improve vascular reactivity, the ability of your blood vessels to change their diameter so more oxygen can reach the brain, thereby increasing mental performance and alertness. For a delicious and healthy treat, try a small piece of dark chocolate right after lunch and see how that helps you perform in the afternoon.[7]

1% TIP: CHOOSE POWER FUEL

The food we consume has a significant impact on the neurotransmitters in our brain that influence our level of energy, alertness, and focus. Eat a dose of carbohydrate and you will need a nap. Eat a dose of high protein and you will feel alert and energized. Choose one of the nutrient-dense foods from the lists on these pages and add it to your meals today.

PRACTICE FOCUS

During Power Work, you must focus to the best of your ability. Mindfulness training is a great first step on the path to increased focus. Mindfulness is an awareness of the world around you in the here and now. Practicing it involves simply taking time every day to put yourself in a location where you're completely undistracted and focusing on one thing. You can recite a mantra, count your breaths, or simply focus on your breathing. Anytime you

---

7   Lorenzo Loffredo, Ludovica Perri, Elisa Catasca, Pasquale Pignatelli, Monica Brancorsini, Cristina Nocella, Elena De Falco, Simona Bartimoccia, Giacomo Frati, Roberto Carnevale, and Francesco Violi, "Dark Chocolate Acutely Improves Walking Autonomy in Patients with Peripheral Artery Disease," *Journal of the American Heart Association* 3, no. 4 (2014): 3:e001072, https://doi.org/10.1161/JAHA.114.001072.

notice your mind wandering, bring it back to that one task. This is done without judgment—there is no good or bad. You are practicing living in the moment and controlling your attention.

With practice and with time, your mindfulness training will begin to elicit remarkable results. After eight weeks of regular meditation, the neurons and tissues inside the brain responsible for helping us stay focused grow. You will start to notice when you are distracted, which sounds simple but is a challenge to most of us. It will put a stop to ruminating thoughts and help you to stay in the moment, which is critical to performing at your best.

Mindfulness can present a cart-and-horse conundrum for some people. They think they don't have enough time to practice mindfulness because they are so overwhelmed and stressed. Yet just the act of doing it helps us feel more centered and in control, which leads to better focus and increased efficiency.

This is another area of our lives where technology can be part of the solution. There are many tools available to help you incorporate mindfulness into your routine. Check out apps such as Headspace and Calm. Another option is the aforementioned Muse, which is an app that works with a headband that picks up brain activity. While wearing it, the user hears water gently crashing on the waves on the beach. As soon as the mind begins to wander, the band picks up the mental activity and changes the sound to storms. The stormy sounds are the user's cue to refocus. Once the user goes more than thirty seconds with no change in brain activity, the sound changes to birds tweeting and points are awarded.

1% TIP: TRAIN YOUR BRAIN TO FOCUS

Use mindfulness and mediation techniques to improve your brain's ability to focus. You can use an app such as Headspace, Calm, or Muse. Or you can just plan to take time out of your day to pause, connect to your breathing, and be in the moment. Do this regularly over the course of several weeks, and you can improve your focus.

90/90/1

Robin Sharma, the leadership speaker best known for his *The Monk Who Sold His Ferrari* book series, is the brainchild behind the 90/90/1 rule, which urges people to spend ninety minutes a day for ninety days in a row working on their number one task. It can be a work project, a fitness goal, a family matter, or any other activity you consider most important at the time. You set aside time every single day to engage with what matters most, and at the end of the ninety days, you have a clear sense of what you were able to accomplish.

I often share this with audiences at my speaking engagements to remind them of the importance of spending critical time every day completely undistracted. I ask them if they can look back at the last month of their lives and really remember what they did. Most cannot. People feel busy because they are constantly jumping from task to task, putting out fires, rather than doing their most important work. Devoting specific time to it each day, without distraction, can help you hone in on your goals with real clarity and purpose.

Research shows ninety minutes is typically what the brain can handle before becoming tired, but if it seems like too much for you at first, you can test yourself to see what works best. Set a timer, begin working on a task, and see if you can go for thirty minutes without getting distracted or moving on to something else. Do that for as long as you feel comfortable, then build up on it with fifteen-minute increments until you reach ninety minutes.

GET INTO FLOW

Have you ever been working diligently at a task, then looked at the clock and been shocked at how much time has passed? Do you feel yourself getting into "the zone" when engaging in an activity you not only excel at but also enjoy? That magical state is called flow. When you establish a state of flow, your energy rises and your work becomes easier to accomplish. It helps you reach your greatest potential.

Flow is not the same as doing something mindlessly. It is a very deliberate practice. Imagine a golfer on the driving range smacking ball, after ball, after ball. He is in a rhythm, and there's nothing interfering with it. He is relaxed, but his actions are deliberate. He is in a state of flow where he can execute his task to the best of his ability.

There are four prerequisites for entering this magical flow state, the first and most important of which is the ability to eliminate all distractions. When you are distracted or attempting to "multitask," you have no chance of getting into flow. Flow is all about single-mindedness. It requires a commitment to staying on task. If you are getting notifications or allowing others to disturb you, your chances of getting into flow are zero.

The second prerequisite for flow is reaching the proper activation level. The Yerkes-Dodson law states that at low activation levels—when you don't care or are tired, bored, or not engaged—your performance is very poor. The same effect happens at high activation levels, when you are nervous, tense, anxious, and stressed. In the middle, when you are activated properly, you are engaged, focused, and excited. You are in a perfect state to activate all your potential at the same time.

Third, you must have a challenge. If the task you're doing is too easy, it won't drive you enough to get into flow. You want to be engaging in something tough but possible for you to accomplish. It should be something slightly beyond your comfort zone.

Fourth, you must be able to control and monitor your emotions. If you are sad, scared, nervous, stressed, or bored, you must address those feeling before attempting to do your best work, as they can prohibit you from entering a flow state. You must put yourself into the proper emotional space to activate flow. The easiest way to do so is to remember previous times you felt flow. Everyone can identify a few times in their lives when they've been in it. While it might seem to happen by accident or at random, the flow state is actually something that can be entered into deliberately.

When you can remember times when you've been at your best, you can remember the emotions you felt and try to replicate the feeling. For example, if you notice you're too nervous, you can do deep breathing to calm yourself down. If you're bored, you can visualize the dream you're trying to accomplish to make yourself feel more excited.

Because we do our best work in this flow state, we all should make it our personal goal to get into flow every single day. When you are in a state of flow, time goes by quickly. You are at your best and more present, which makes you more productive and the workday seem to go faster. Pick the task most important for you—whether it's your workout, being with your family, a work project, anything—and let your mind commit to it fully. If you start with a mindfulness exercise and stay focused, flow will come.

> ### 1% TIP: FIND YOUR FLOW
>
> Pick a task that is important to you—in any area of your life—and commit to achieving a state of flow while engaged in it. A state of flow has four qualities: (1) no distractions, (2) a level of activation that is neither too low (boredom or apathy) nor too high (stress and anxiousness), (3) a challenge that is slightly beyond your comfort zone, and (4) deliberate control of emotions to enable complete immersion in the task.

PREPARE OTHERS

The last step to ensuring an ideal Power Work routine is informing those close to you about your new approach. The important people in your world need to understand the importance of your Power Work time. Explain that while it allows you to get home earlier and be more productive, it also means you can't check every text the instant it arrives. Explain your schedule so they know when you are on task or available.

Have a system in place so you can be reached in case of an

emergency. Give them an emergency number to call, or edit the contacts in your phone so certain people can get through in emergency calls. Remember, overcommunication is always better. When everyone fully understands what you're doing and why, they won't see you as simply disappearing, and everyone will feel better about it.

CHAPTER 4

Master the Evening: Recovery and Regeneration

When work is done, it's time to focus on preparing yourself for rest and recovery so you can again be at your best the next day. As an example, let's assume you finish your morning routine by 7:00 a.m. and are at your desk ready to start the workday by 8:00 a.m. With Power Work, you are done earlier than normal. So how should you spend the rest of your day?

Early afternoon to 5:00 p.m. can now be time you spend on yourself, however you choose to do so. You can spend it networking, holding meetings, learning new skills, or researching topics of interest. You can spend it getting a massage and unwinding from the productive morning. As long as this time does not become wasted, the possibilities for its use are endless.

From 5:00 to 6:00 p.m., you can head home, spend time with family, and begin to prepare for an evening of recovery and recharging.

GET THE MOST OUT OF THE EVENING

The evening routine is just as important as the morning routine. This is when you regenerate and set yourself up for an amazing sleep. Your quality of sleep depends greatly on what you do in the evening.

If you are the kind of person whose mind races before sleep, thinking about the next day, take time well before your evening routine to plan and prepare for anything on your agenda. Look at your next day and prepare for any important calls, review any notes, plan your Power Work time, or do any other thing you need to do so you can put all that thinking aside until the next day. You might do this at the end of your workday, or perhaps after dinner. Do not let it interfere with the time you will devote to relaxing and recharging in the evening.

The most important step to take when you begin your evening routine is avoiding devices and screens for at least an hour before you go to sleep, ninety minutes preferably.

This gives your brain time to get quiet and calm in preparation for rest. Bombarding it with images and noise so close to its period of recovery keeps it from fully shutting down when you need it to. Use this time to instead relax with your partner, enjoy a glass of wine, take a walk, simply sit and talk, play a sport, read a book, or learn a new skill.

Do whatever best helps you unwind. For me, it's a hot bath with Epsom salts. The warm water is calming while the salts help my body recover from the day's workout. I follow my bath with a quick cold shower. Switching between temperatures triggers the release of melatonin, which helps me to fall asleep quickly.

I follow this with a short bit of meditation to relax my mind, then some light fiction reading, which gives my brain a rest from all the things that have been demanding its attention during the course of the day. Difficult as it may be, I highly recommend avoiding any TV news before bed. To me, the stimulation we get from the constant news cycle today is like nothing we've ever seen before. Those programs tend to keep me awake and set my mind racing again.

My routine takes about an hour, and it is well worth it, as I sleep deeply and well. If I jump right into bed, I'm restless. I wake up in the middle of the night, and I can't fall back asleep again. It's important to create a barrier between the day and sleep, so the mind can calm and we can fall asleep deeply and quickly. This crucial practice allows us to relax, rejuvenate, and regenerate properly.

When need be, adjust your schedule to account for proper sleep needs. For instance, if you are going to an event and won't be home until 11:00 p.m., switch your routine to start a little later the next day. Do not schedule anything the next morning that disrupts your goal of seven to eight hours of sleep. Do not deprive your body and mind of its recovery and regeneration time.

The key here, as it is in so many things pertaining to focus, is to do this all deliberately. Plan for it, and remove all guesswork. This is what leads to success for many high-achieving people, whether they be entrepreneurs or athletes. They plan, plan, plan their days and routines. Nothing is haphazard. This allows them to both be at their best and be prepared mentally and physically to take on any unforeseen challenges the day might bring.

1% TIP: PROTECT YOUR FINAL HOUR BEFORE BED

How you spend the sixty to ninety minutes before bed has a substantial effect on the quality and duration of your night's sleep. Establish a ritual that allows you to wind down rather than jumping directly into bed, and do all you can to consistently stick to this routine. Avoid devices during this time, engage in relaxing activities such as walking, talking, or taking a bath, and finish with some brief meditation or some light fiction in bed.

NO EXCUSES

Many people reading this might think, *This all sounds great, but who has the time?* The most common excuse for not changing behavior is, "I'm too busy." If this is you, I challenge you to really think about how you are spending your time.

One of the biggest forms of distraction is TV. The average North American spends between thirty and thirty-eight hours a week watching TV. Kids spend even more.

If you are watching TV thirty hours a week, you have time to devote to morning and evening routines. You have time to work out, eat right, and get all the rest and relaxation your body needs—you are just choosing to spend that time doing other things. I realize that I am an extreme in that I don't own a TV. If I work out two hours a day for three days a week, that's six hours. That still leaves me with twenty-four more hours a week than the person watching thirty hours of TV.

TV is just one example of how people waste time. If you were to track your time for an entire week, writing down everything you do in fifteen-minute increments, you would discover the other ways you are giving more time to the things that don't really matter. If you can reallocate that time for something important, you will be amazed how much quicker you reach your goals. If you want to be great, whether at business, fitness, as a parent, or as a spouse, you must give of your time, effort, and energy. Once you do, you will reach your potential.

Ask yourself, "Do my actions mask my ambitions?" It's important you contemplate what you want out of life— what *you* want, not what others want. If you want to build an empire, you probably don't have time to be binge-watching a show. If you have ambitions of building a world-class business, wasting endless hours scrolling through social media isn't an option. You must do the work. Make sure what you are actually doing reflects your goals and dreams. If they are not one and the same, look within yourself and figure out a way to bring them into alignment.

DON'T WAIT FOR CRISIS

We have evolved into a state of digital distraction over the last five to fifteen years where we can't even identify what is causing the underlying angst, anxiety, or depression so many of us feel. Never allowing ourselves to shut off contributes directly to a decline in mental health, yet many of us don't realize it until it is too late. The damage has been done, and all we hope to do is undo it to the best of our ability.

The only time most of us ever make big changes is when we are finally at a crisis point. But if you wait until that crisis point, you or your company might be beyond saving. Crisis can manifest in many different ways. The only way to avoid it as best you can is by prioritizing your own health and well-being. You must make a commitment to a better lifestyle so you can perform at a world-class level and make short-term sacrifices to better yourself in future. This thinking applies to us as individuals and to our organizations as well. We need to be aware and proactive.

We all are working in a way that doesn't work for us anymore. You might feel stuck in a mindset of "that's just the way it is," but you cannot afford to think that way. You must change before you have a personal health crisis, get divorced, lose your company, or go bankrupt. You must disrupt yourself and disrupt your own company before your devotion to an archaic way of working takes its toll.

It's not about breaking what's not broken. It's about shining a light on what is broken and the impact it's having on our lives and those of future generations.

There are many ways to approach life slightly differently and slowly make changes to improve your life. You can change your habits one step at a time. As you do, you will begin to realize the benefits, and changing other behaviors will become easier. You will feel better, work better, and live better. The sooner you start, the sooner you will see the change.

Personal Mastery Checklist

OVERVIEW

In a world of constant distractions and activities, unhealthy food, and habits that drain our energy, we can all benefit from taking a step back to assess how we live. By setting up our days to help us be as focused as possible as often as possible, we can live happy, healthy, productive, and successful lives.

THE QUIZ

Answer the questions below to assess how well you have set up your life for optimal focus, wellness, and productivity. Your responses will assist you in identifying simple changes you can make to get more out of your time and fully enjoy your life and work.

DIRECTIONS

Select the answer that best matches your current behavior. Your responses give you a sense of how you are supporting your ability to achieve the Focus Effect. Add up your scores at the end to see how you are doing. You can make minor changes by addressing one question at a time. Then come back in a couple of months to take the quiz again and see how your focus has improved!

1. CAN YOU AVOID STOPPING AND STARTING DURING A TASK?

- Always (5 points)
- Yup (4 points)
- Pretty much (3 points)
- Sort of (2 points)
- Not really (1 point)
- Never (0 points)

Recommendations: Before you begin a task, turn off all notifications and set aside any distractions so that once you have started, you can see the task through to completion.

Rationale: If we task-switch and jump back and forth between activities, different parts of the brain are activated. As a result, blood flow has to move from one location to another, and that takes time. You activate one part of the brain and deliver nutrients to it, and then you shut that part down and open up another. Therefore, multitasking is actually a highly inefficient process for the brain. It simply doesn't work that way.

2. DO YOU FOLLOW A MORNING ROUTINE THAT SETS YOU UP FOR SUCCESS?

- Always (5 points)
- Yup (4 points)
- Pretty much (3 points)
- Sort of (2 points)
- Not really (1 point)
- Never (0 points)

Recommendations: Have a checklist—either in mind or written down—that you follow every morning so that you go through a deliberate routine that will set you up with energy and focus for the day ahead. Include on the checklist a morning affirmation, brief meditation, or moment of mindfulness, Power Fuel, and some exercise to get your brain going.

Rationale: Research has demonstrated that the mental and physical activities a person engages in first thing in the morning can shape their attitude, level of alertness, and focus for the entire day. Affirmations put you in a positive mental space. Mindfulness clears out negative thoughts.

High-protein and high-fiber foods set us on the right track for consistent energy all day. Physical activity first thing in the morning helps to optimize brain growth and memory. And keeping away from the mental distraction of dealing with emails will help you put off those demands on your mind until you are ready.

3. DO YOU IDENTIFY YOUR MOST PRODUCTIVE TIME OF DAY AND USE THIS TIME FOR POWER WORK?

- Always (5 points)
- Yup (4 points)
- Pretty much (3 points)
- Sort of (2 points)
- Not really (1 point)
- Never (0 points)

Recommendations: Monitor your energy levels throughout the day to determine when you are at your most effective. Then set yourself up to spend uninterrupted time working on your most important tasks. Shut off all notifications, clear your schedule, avoid email, and let everyone know that you are offline during this time. Tackle the work in ninety-minute blocks with thirty minutes of active, healthy rest between work sessions. You can then attend to less-demanding tasks at a time of day when you are in a lower energy state and less is demanded of you.

Rationale: By optimizing the amount you get done on your most important tasks at a time when you are at your best, you can radically improve your overall productivity.

4. DO YOU TAKE ACTIVE HEALTHY BREAKS?

- Always (5 points)
- Yup (4 points)
- Pretty much (3 points)
- Sort of (2 points)
- Not really (1 point)
- Never (0 points)

Recommendations: In between blocks of work, rather than sitting on your phone or eating a sugary snack, make a deliberate effort to get up and move around, whether that is taking a walk or doing something simple such as power yoga. Eat some nutritious food high in healthy fats, proteins, and fiber that will give you sustained fuel. Take time to give your mind a break, either through a mindfulness activity or just letting your mind be free from focus and effort.

Rationale: The human brain is not particularly energy efficient, so after ninety minutes of focused work, its effectiveness declines rapidly. Exercise and nutritious food, along with thirty minutes of time for your brain to recover by not focusing on a task, will restore this energy for another ninety minutes of top-notch effort.

5. DO YOU SHUT OFF NOTIFICATIONS AND REMOVE DISTRACTIONS?

- Always (5 points)
- Yup (4 points)
- Pretty much (3 points)
- Sort of (2 points)
- Not really (1 point)
- Never (0 points)

Recommendations: When you are working on an important task or in a meeting, put your devices in do-not-disturb mode and ensure that no one can interrupt you.

Rationale: Given the importance of starting a task and sticking with it, you have to put structures in place to ensure you are not interrupted. This begins with being deliberate about when you are going to focus on your correspondence and when you are going to work on projects or be in meetings so that you can give your full attention to the task at hand.

6. DO YOU USE POSITIVE SELF-TALK TO MOTIVATE YOURSELF?

- Always (5 points)
- Yup (4 points)
- Pretty much (3 points)
- Sort of (2 points)

- Not really (1 point)
- Never (0 points)

Recommendations: Make use of positive affirmations that you say out loud to yourself at the beginning of the day and also prior to a challenging meeting or task so that you are in the headspace to succeed.

Rationale: Research indicates that a positive attitude has a strong impact on performance, so by using this technique regularly, you can ensure you are at your best. By entering into a situation clear about your intentions and sure of your ability to achieve the goal, you will be focused on success and proceed with confidence.

7. DO YOU EAT NUTRIENT-DENSE FOODS THAT WILL FUEL YOUR PERFORMANCE?

- Always (5 points)
- Yup (4 points)
- Pretty much (3 points)
- Sort of (2 points)
- Not really (1 point)
- Never (0 points)

Recommendations: Ensure your diet is packed with foods that contribute to health, productivity, energy, and well-being. Nutrient-dense foods optimal for Power Fuel include organic grass-fed meats, cold-water fish, black beans, berries, avocado, raw nuts, seeds, eggs (particularly omelets with greens), coconut, kale, and ginger.

Rationale: The food we consume has a substantial effect on the neurotransmitters in our brains. For example, if we eat foods higher in protein than carbohydrates, we increase the number of neurotransmitters that help us concentrate and stay focused. If we eat foods higher in carbohydrates than protein, we increase the neurotransmitters that widen our focus and help us to relax. Your performance today, your overall feeling of energy and alertness, and your long-term health all rely on consistently eating great food.

8. DO YOU PLAN YOUR FOOD?

- Always (5 points)
- Yup (4 points)
- Pretty much (3 points)
- Sort of (2 points)
- Not really (1 point)
- Never (0 points)

Recommendations: Map out your food plan for the week and the day so that you avoid grazing or scrambling around to find some fuel when you are tired, busy, or stressed.

Rationale: Unhealthy food choices are all around us, and more often than not, if we do not have a plan to ensure we have access to the nutrient-dense foods we need for consistent fuel and ongoing alertness, we are likely to start eating foods that will make us tired, distracted, and ineffective.

9. DO YOU EXERCISE REGULARLY?

- Always (5 points)
- Yup (4 points)
- Pretty much (3 points)
- Sort of (2 points)
- Not really (1 point)
- Never (0 points)

Recommendations: Make plans to ensure you get regular exercise, including planning for both a workout of some kind and also for simple movement such as a walk or yoga.

Rationale: Movement improves mental function and also addresses any issues you might have with anxiety or depression. Exercise also activates the part of your brain associated with creativity and problem solving. It makes us sharper and more capable of concentration.

10. DO YOU PRACTICE MINDFULNESS?

- Always (5 points)

- Yup (4 points)
- Pretty much (3 points)
- Sort of (2 points)
- Not really (1 point)
- Never (0 points)

Recommendations: Use mindfulness or meditation to train your brain to focus and develop habits for clearing your mind of clutter and stress. You can begin slowly by just taking five minutes to focus on your breathing and move from there to mindfulness apps such as Muse or Calm or by getting some training in basic meditation techniques.

Rationale: We get better at what we do repeatedly. If you work at training your brain to focus and control thoughts, you can rapidly improve your focus. After eight weeks of regular meditation, the neurons and tissues inside the brain responsible for helping us stay focused start to grow. You will begin to find that you are aware of when you are distracted, which will enable you to manage your focus more effectively. You will also develop the capacity to stop needless mental looping and stay in the moment, which are both critical to performing at your best.

11. DO YOU FOLLOW A STRUCTURED ROUTINE FOR THE FINAL HOUR BEFORE BED?

- Always (5 points)

- Yup (4 points)
- Pretty much (3 points)
- Sort of (2 points)
- Not really (1 point)
- Never (0 points)

Recommendations: Create a pre-bed routine that helps your mind wind down from the day and avoids stimulation. Avoid devices during this time; instead, take a calming walk, have a glass of wine with your partner, or just take some time for mindfulness. Also, consider reading some light fiction once you are in bed, which will help your mind to relax and calm you down so you are ready for a long and deep sleep. Also, if you have a lot to get done, try to get a solid list written out before your final hour so that those tasks are not on your mind while you are giving your brain a break.

Rationale: Quality sleep is one of the most important determinants of focus, and the final hour before bed has a significant impact on our sleep. Our brains need time to wind down from the day, so you need to protect that time by avoiding stimulation.

12. HAVE YOU INFORMED EVERYONE IN YOUR LIFE ABOUT YOUR APPROACH TO COMMUNICATION?

- Always (5 points)

- Yup (4 points)
- Pretty much (3 points)
- Sort of (2 points)
- Not really (1 point)
- Never (0 points)

Recommendations: Make sure that everyone in your life understands that there will be times in the day when you are not to be disturbed and will not be responding to them. Arrange for a system in the event that an actual emergency arises (but they rarely do).

Rationale: Letting people know about how you are going to approach your work sets their expectations and ensures that you can actually focus on what you are trying to accomplish. When everyone fully understands what you're doing and why, they won't see you as simply disappearing, and everyone will feel better about it.

TOTAL SCORE

40+ points:
You are living the dream! You have set up your life to optimize your focus and ensure you perform at your best most of the time.

20–39 points:

You are getting there. Keep tweaking your approach to find more areas for focus in your life.

0–19 points:

You have made a start, but there is work to be done. Pick one item from the quiz above and work on it this week. After you have made some changes in that area, you can come back and focus on another area for improvement.

PART 2

Work Mastery

. . . .

The performer who focuses the best wins the most.
—CHAD REMPEL

CHAPTER 5

The Cult of Busyness in the Workplace

Not long ago, two consultants from a large firm with which we do business asked to meet with me to pitch me on using their services. They came into the AMJ boardroom, sat across from me, and began speaking.

As soon as one would start to speak, the other would begin texting and emailing while his colleague spoke. When the first one stopped speaking, the other would chime in, and the first one would reach for his phone.

It was beyond rude. It was absurd that I was giving these men any of my time. I found myself thinking, *When did this become acceptable?*

"Hey, guys," I said. "You are obviously way too busy for me. Why don't you come back when you're not so busy?"

They were shocked.

I said, "Look, both of you are clearly distracted."

They apologized and explained they were in the middle of another important project.

"Not to worry," I said. "Go work on your project. Come back when you're ready to give me your full attention."

Needless to say, we never met again, but it caused me to really question when this kind of behavior became OK. It's happening all the time, even within my own company. To curb it, I have implemented a process whereby every time we gather for meetings in our boardrooms, we put our cell phones into a basket. Loved ones who might need to reach them urgently are instructed to call my assistant. Because true emergencies are thankfully few and far between, this practice is rarely necessary.

The story is just one example of how we all have become numb to the presence of distraction in our lives. The consultants who could not focus on our meeting saw nothing wrong with what they were doing. The Cult of Busyness has given people permission to act in this manner. They try to do as much as they can at all times. Their focus is divided among so many different things that no one person or task ever gets full attention. We see it commonly at service counters, stores, and other workplaces where we find ourselves waiting while someone behind the counter or reception desk is texting, oblivious to us.

Both focus and paying close attention are required if you want to reach your full potential. If you are trying to make a difference in the world by creating something, running a successful business, improving your job skills, or simply being a great family member or friend, the single most important thing you can do is focus your attention on what matters most.

THE EIGHT-HOUR WORKDAY RELIC

Feeding into the Cult of Busyness is the long-standing belief that a productive workday must last, at the very least, eight hours. The concept of the eight-hour workday started with the Industrial Revolution. Ford Motor Company advanced the idea in 1914, when the company scaled back its forty-eight-hour work week to curb accidents.

While there is plenty of research about why certain work structures were put into place in terms of processes, there is no information about why the eight-hour workday still makes sense. We have all learned to use it as a guideline in our businesses for centuries, but no one understands exactly why.

Because we've been doing this for so long, eight hours has become the minimally acceptable measure of work. If you hold a salaried management position and work forty hours a week, you are meeting the bare minimum expectations. The unspoken expectation is you should be the first one in the office every morning and the last one to leave every night. Otherwise, you're seen as a slacker.

When I began my career as a banker, I was that person. I worked sixty to seventy hours a week and was the first one in and last one out. This was a poor measurement of performance and skill. In retrospect, I realize that lifestyle didn't make me any more productive; it just made me get up earlier and get home later. I spent plenty of time twiddling my thumbs. I doubt I actually worked forty of those seventy hours. Yet many business leaders today hold firm to the belief that if they worked sixty hours a week when they began their careers, then dammit, everyone behind them should suffer the same fate.

I am a fan of hard work, and there are certainly times in our careers when extra demands require extra time, but it is not sustainable long term if we have any hope of living a balanced life. Many leaders of the newest and fastest-growing companies are far more focused on working smarter, not harder or longer. Balance and lifestyle have become important hallmarks of these companies. When I was beginning my career, everyone believed the early bird gets the worm; today, the early bird might get the worm, but the second mouse gets the cheese.

ADAPTING TO A CHANGING WORLD

Our society is in the midst of a technological revolution, which will require just as much of a change in the way we think and work as the previous revolution did. The sooner we can absolve ourselves of this antiquated way of approaching the workday, the sooner we will be able to create greater opportunities for growth for ourselves and for our companies.

When you eliminate distraction from your day, there is no need to be chained to a desk for endless hours. We have seen many examples of successful companies that have implemented five-, six-, and seven-hour workdays, with flexible hours and have shown far more daily productivity than the traditional eight-hour workday. Heck, some companies would be happy to go from ten- to twelve-hour workdays down to eight.

I recently got into a lively discussion with a lawyer. We were debating the need to work associate lawyers fresh out of school for sixty, seventy, even eighty-plus hours a week. His argument was, "That's how we had to do it when I started. It's how we see what they are made of." Really? If we look at the four emerging giants of industry—Facebook, Google, Amazon, and Apple—companies whose revenue, growth, and profitability are beyond impressive, we won't find such an archaic attitude toward work hours. It's often the opposite—they are attracting and retaining the brightest talent in the world precisely because they offer something more than being "worked to the bone."

Many traditional businesses, including law firms, banks, insurance companies, and even my own company, are going to have to reengineer our workplace environment, structure, and experience if we want to be around in twenty years. Given the choice, why would a millennial choose long, unhealthy work weeks over companies with more enlightened views about work hours such as the four aforementioned giants?

The key to success is not a longer day with more hours—it is a day with focus. The goal of our book and our program is to show other employees and employers that a day absent of distraction and centered on focus is far more productive than a long tedious day chained to a desk. As an employer, why wouldn't you want employees who are happier doing work in less time versus people who are miserable all day? As an employee, if you want to become a star who gets noticed and promoted, do it by becoming more focused, less distracted, and far more productive. Focus fuels performance.

LEAVING THE CULT OF BUSYNESS TAKES FOCUS

Distractions must be set aside during on-task time. When you are working, you are working. When you are not working, you are recovering and regenerating so you can do your best work again the next day.

I began applying this practice in my own life last year. I was working on a book, *The Ripple Effect*, which is now available.[8] For about a year, I was working on it in what I thought was a diligent manner, but I wasn't making much progress. The writing was not great, and I knew I could do better.

I had written two versions of the book. Both were OK but not great. I was trying to do it little by little here and there, and it was showing in the writing. I realized my attention was too widespread. I had multiple other balls in the air and was always thinking about the next project, even when I was sitting down to write.

I decided to drop everything and make the book my top priority. I assigned importance to it. I realized I needed to take a short-term hit for a long-term gain. I blocked

---

8   Greg Wells, *The Ripple Effect* (Toronto: HarperCollins Canada, 2017).

three months off my calendar. I did not take on any other projects or business ventures. I refused to schedule any speaking engagement or unrelated meetings.

I devised a schedule and followed it every day. I got up in the morning, worked out, went to the coffee shop, got a double espresso, went to my office, and worked for five hours completely undistracted. I dropped deep into the content and continually made progress.

I was able to produce a book I am extremely proud of in just three months. It went on to become a national best-seller in Canada. It was all because I was able to create an environment, a routine, and a strategy around doing my best work at a critical time.

When you give your tasks your undivided attention, you are able to produce higher quality work in less time. There is no logic to sitting at a desk for a designated amount of time if the work you are completing is not the best representation of your abilities.

WORDS OF WISDOM: EIGHT-TIME
OLYMPIAN IAN MILLAR

Eight-time Olympic equestrian Ian Millar of Canada harnesses the power of focus every time he's in the saddle.

His sport is both physically and psychologically demanding, and he must remain in control at all times. He must be activated but not tense. When the horse senses tension, it becomes nervous and can't do what it needs to do.

"There's a total mind connection between the rider and the horse," Ian says. "Stress levels are intimately linked. Just having a thought impacts the horse. Managing the self is absolutely critical."

The key to achieving the balance, he says, is focus. It is something he practices until it becomes automatic. He has worked his entire career learning how to master it.

He begins by blocking out any thoughts of the past and future and living only in the present.

During the Nations Cup Hong Kong competition before the Beijing Olympics, Ian was the last rider of four. He needed to ride a clean performance to tie the Americans and qualify for the Olympics. On his way to the course, his teammates were trying to help by giving him advice. Ian could tell they were nervous, and he knew he could not allow that kind of energy to affect him or his horse. He relied on his practice with focus and was able to ignore them completely. He blocked them out, focused entirely on his performance, and went on to compete in Beijing.

The relationship between rider and horse can also apply to leader and team, salesperson and client, speaker and audience, and many others. Your ability to focus keeps you and everyone around you performing at peak potential.

Just as Ian does this, so can you with enough practice.

As Ian likes to say, "I never give up until I succeed, and I never give up."

CHAPTER 6

The Focused Workplace

With the power of focus comes freedom. No longer must you adhere to an archaic work schedule of eight, nine, or ten-plus hours a day. You are more efficient because you possess a higher ability to execute tasks while free from distractions. When you apply those skills in the workplace, you can begin to make changes that will improve every aspect of your life.

The work-life balance program we initiated at our company was designed with the goal of creating a six- or seven-hour workday. We implemented it with the intention of putting the ideas about life and work balance we'd extensively researched into practice. The pilot involved a number of employees of AMJ Campbell Van Lines in Toronto and lasted for three months, although many of the practices taught during that time have become long-standing. The results have been amazing. Employees are happier, more engaged, more productive, and even healthier—we saw a significant decrease in the number of sick days taken. All of this showed us these methods have true value that can and will work.

**1% TIP: CHANGE YOUR THINKING
ABOUT THE WORKDAY**

When a working environment is shaped by an emphasis on the value of employees' time at work rather than a fixed notion of how long they work, good things happen. By implementing a range of structures that radically improve productivity, workplaces can decrease the workday and ensure healthy and happy employees who have a reasonable work-life balance while improving the performance of the company.

A disclaimer: It's OK if a six- or seven-hour day does not seem reasonable to you. For some, even an eight-hour workday would be an improvement. Cater the following advice and guidance to fit your needs and your schedule. The shorter workday example is just one way to think about using your newfound focus to improve your productivity while reducing your work hours. Our goal was to produce incentives for employees to become more focused and create a healthier environment.

Remember, it's not just about the hours you are working.

It's about structuring the time you are working in a way that's healthier than what you were doing before. It's about living a very different life. It's not simply about volume; it's about high performance. I liken it to how we trained athletes twenty years ago versus today. Back then, whoever got the most mileage in and didn't get injured was the one who made the Olympics. Today, it's much more holistic. It's about training, performing, recovering, regenerating, and staying healthy. Because of this new approach, athletes are continuing to break world records and enjoying much longer careers. They used to be done in their early twenties, whereas now we're seeing people with medals in their thirties and forties. It's almost doubled the amount of time someone can be an elite athlete. They're healthier, they're higher performing, and I believe they're all much happier.

A SPRINT, NOT A MARATHON

By considering work as a series of sprints interspersed with recovery, we can perform at the higher level, get more done in less time, and be healthier altogether. We need to structure our days in a way so that we are waking up, setting ourselves up for a great day, performing optimally, recovering and regenerating, and then having a fantastic time with our families, exercising, doing activities we love, reading, learning, and doing all the things that make up an incredible life.

If companies can get on board with this thinking, their people are going to be healthier, happier, higher performing, and enjoying an overall better environment. One of the most important things we witnessed during the implementation of our program is the change in people's moods at the end of the day. They used to just finish their work and leave. Now they take the time to say good-night to one another. They say, "Hey, have a great rest of your day. See you later." That never happened before. People would finish their work, and it was like, "Just get me out of here." Now it's like almost as if they're offering a thank-you at the end of the day. It's just one example of how these changes can lead to very profound side effects.

ASSAULTED WITH INFORMATION

The incessant nature of information we live with every day takes a potentially dangerous toll on all of us. The feeling of being overwhelmed can result in several physiological responses, none of which are good. It is believed that the average person today is exposed to more information in one month than our great-great-grandparents were exposed to in a lifetime. With instant news, social media, and a constant barrage of information, it is a recipe for information overload.

From a leadership vantage point, I watch as employees try to cope with the stress of being turned on all the time.

They are active from morning to night with no breaks. The burnout we see today is different than what we've seen in the past. Before, we could say, "I've been working on this project for six months, and it's burned me out." It was the length and scope of the work that drained us. Today's burnout is fueled by anxiety. People are bombarded by so many mini-stresses; they can't identify just one as the cause of burnout. It's death by a thousand cuts, or in this case, a thousand emails.

Because of this never-ending onslaught, we have modified our behavior in an attempt to stay informed up to the second. We have learned to communicate in 144 characters or fewer, which is great for efficiency and awful for our mental function. It is robbing us of our ability to focus. The average North American today never reads a book past age forty. It's not because they're not interested—they simply can't stay focused on anything that demands more of their attention than the average social media post. Our brains are not wired to receive so many messages instantaneously, and we're suffering for it.

The result is reduced productivity and engagement, both at the office and at home. We are compromising our ability to do our work and our ability to have a healthy home life, because the lines between the two are blurred. As a result, we're at home when we're at work, and we're at work when we're at home. This leads us to feel like we lack sufficient time to adequately perform either role. In reality, if we eliminated distraction and truly devoted ourselves to one role at a time, our performance at both would sky rocket. We would have so much more happiness because we wouldn't feel so conflicted all the time.

THE MYTH OF MULTITASKING

All this role juggling forces us to live in a constant state of playing catch-up. We try to stay ahead of the game by multitasking, but this only causes us to become even more distracted. Just think about the last month of your life. Can you actually remember what you've accomplished or is it just a blur? If you're like most people, you try to do too much at once and therefore end up not producing anything of real value.

Our brains are truly not capable of multitasking. We cannot do two things at once. We might think we are tackling more than one activity simultaneously when in reality, all we are doing is switching back and forth from one task to another. Every time we switch, we lose focus and have to reorient our brains, and that does not happen as quickly as we think. Research shows it takes an average of fifteen minutes to reorient yourself to a primary task after a distraction, which results in a 40 percent drop in productivity.[9]

9   Paul Atchley, "You Can't Multitask, So Stop Trying," *Harvard Business Review*, December 21, 2010, https://hbr.org/2010/12/you-cant-multi-task-so-stop-tr.

Let's say you are doing something on your computer and speaking on the phone at the same time. Those tasks require attention from separate parts of the brain: your thinking center and your audio-processing center. These centers are not working at the same time. When you try to use both simultaneously, you end up using neither. Your brain is not focused on what's happening on the computer, nor is it focused on the phone call. By trying to spread your attention among so many things, you're not giving any one thing your full focus.

This is what the medical community refers to as a "task-switching cost." Multitasking costs a great deal of energy in the brain. Oxygen and blood flow must be delivered to any part of the brain for it to work. Moving oxygen and blood flow from one part to another so quickly and frequently is dramatically inefficient.

I experienced this firsthand several years ago when I

thought I would be clever and get two twenty-four-inch computer screens in my office. I could have my emails, messages, Google, calendar, and whatever else I wanted open at all times. I would flip back and forth between it all, and I thought I was being highly efficient. I soon realized it actually slowed me down. I found it to be dizzying, and it caused a noticeable lack of focus. Bouncing around from task to task did not give my brain enough time to retain information. I could not remember things as clearly as I did before. I felt stressed out and bombarded.

Today, I have one screen and focus on one task or project at a time. I turn off notices and check emails and messages periodically during the day. I am more focused, less stressed and scattered, and I am far more productive.

We need to learn to single-task, which requires a certain degree of mindfulness. We must choose what activities and tasks are truly worthy of our time and attention, then commit to devoting our full focus to them. When we are with our families, we must be with our families. When we are at work, we must be focused on work.

When our attention is divided among too many things, we are not truly engaged with any one task. According to Gallup Daily tracking, only about one-third of US employees are engaged, meaning they are involved in, enthusiastic about, and committed to their work and workplace. Worldwide, just 13 percent of employees are engaged.[10]

While none of this is good for business, the effect of distraction on our personal well-being can be even more alarming. According to a bebrainfit.com article, "The Cognitive Costs of Multitasking," multitasking "doesn't just slow you down, it also increases the number of mistakes you make. One study found that subjects given three tasks to perform made three times as many errors as those given only two tasks." The article also reports that multitasking hurts cognitive performance and short-term memory and can temporarily reduce IQ by fifteen points.[11]

DO NOT DISTURB

A great first step toward eliminating distractions is stopping the barrage of messages we constantly receive. Silence your phone or put in another room, close any windows on your computer that aren't essential to your work, and disable desktop notifications. This might be difficult at first, but you will likely soon realize you are truly not missing anything of any importance.

10   Annamarie Mann and Jim Harter, "The Worldwide Employee Engagement Crisis," *Gallup*, January 7, 2016, http://news.gallup.com/businessjournal/188033/worldwide-employee-engagement-crisis.aspx.

11   Deane Alban, "The Cognitive Costs of Multitasking," *Be Brain Fit*, https://bebrainfit.com/cognitive-costs-multitasking/.

For most of us, true emergencies happen only a handful of times throughout our lives, and nothing can happen on social media in ninety minutes that we can't catch up on once we're done with our work. If you absolutely have to be reachable, either by family or clients, create a way for them to do so in case of emergency. Otherwise, do your best to remain completely undisturbed when focusing on your tasks. When we implemented this practice into our own work-life balance pilot program, we never once had a problem with an employee being unreachable in an urgent situation.

Your loved ones don't have to feel completely out of the loop because of this. Let those close to you know what your work schedule looks like so they know the appropriate times to reach you. You can even share your calendar with them electronically.

This helps curb our addiction to being instantaneously reactive and instead helps us become deliberately responsive. If you're immediately reactive, you're constantly jumping from task to task with no real purpose or intention. A call comes in and you instantly answer, whether you are in the proper mindset to do so or not. However, if you are deliberately responding, you might choose to ignore that same call. Then, when you are ready, you can take a moment to compose yourself, organize your thoughts, orchestrate a plan, call the person back, and execute the call perfectly. It might be ten minutes later, but you're much more prepared, and therefore, the outcome is better.

If you do miss something, whether it's another business opportunity or a big news story breaking, you must be willing to accept the consequences. True disconnection from distraction is about prioritization of what's important to you. You live with the outcome because you know in your heart you are working on the most important thing in your life, and it's worth it.

1% TIP: ACTIVELY AVOID DISRUPTIONS

Develop systems where you are in "do not disturb" mode and can focus completely on the task, meeting, or activity you are engaged with. Make it clear to people who need access to you that this is what is happening so they know when they will hear back from you, and you won't feel a need to come up for air constantly to respond to them.

Some of the most successful companies of the last ten years are forgoing traditional workplace practices and offering real flexibility. The brightest minds coming out of the top schools are flocking to these positions over traditional nine-to-five jobs.

Google, for example, provides healthy food for its employees in cafeterias located on every floor of the building. The food is marked with green, yellow, or red labels, indicating how healthy it is for you. If you want the ice cream, it's there, but it's in the red section. They also have fresh spices employees can take home to encourage them to cook more. They want their employees to be healthy at work and at home.

Google also requires employees to work on a creative project of their choosing one day a week. It does not have to be related to the employee's actual job. The practice has led to the creation of Google Maps and other useful tools.

The company's employees are also expected to get away from their computers once a week and spend the day working from a tablet or phone. They want their teams to be mobile.

This is just one example of a highly successful company that didn't follow the rules that had been in place since the Industrial Revolution. The founders came up with a lifestyle that worked well for them and has attracted top talent.

People want real balance in their lives. To get it, we have to stop obsessing about the clock. Putting in hours is not important; creating things of value and purpose is.

Thinking this way can inspire you to change the way you

approach every day. It can be exciting and fun. You spend less time sitting at a desk yet end up producing more.

CHAPTER 7

Create the Space

There are several ways you can alter the physical environment to change the way you work. You might not be able to change the state of your building, but you can make small changes to certain workspaces or rooms that make a big difference. You don't have to spend a ton of money to completely change or replace your existing environment—you can work with what you have to create a space more conducive to improved focus.

Many people work at sitting desks, but there are other options. Standing or walking desks are great if you are working on a project that doesn't require you to be isolated. Employees can use those for phone calls or emails. Another option is bar stools at high tables. You can just lean on them and have a conversation.

There are chairs designed to help you move. You can adjust

the arms, the back, and the height throughout the day. In doing so, you actually move a tremendous amount even though you are seated in your chair. Stability balls are another excellent option for seated movement.

I also try, when possible and appropriate, to get away from the desk. I hold walking meetings where participants get to enjoy a few minutes of fresh air outside. Even moving a meeting off site to a local coffee shop can get the blood flowing in a way sitting around a desk never can.

Some progressive companies offer meditation rooms with comfortable chairs and background music. Employees can come in to close their eyes and take a break in a very quiet place. They can work on mindfulness or meditation. This is a great opportunity for companies to provide things such as Muse headbands or other meditation devices for employees to use. I've also been to a workplace that had a music room—a soundproof room with instruments where employees can go to play some music for a little while. If no such space exists, employees can create their own by putting on headphones, positioning their chairs so they are facing away from door, or finding a place in the building—maybe in a warehouse or meeting room—where they can go to disconnect.

Make sure the vending machines in your break spaces offer some healthy options. The typical standard garbage you get in and around office buildings can literally make you sick. Think about what options you can provide so people get the nutrition they need for optimal performance. If possible, provide free healthy snacks to give employees incentives to make better food choices.

Lighting also can play an important role in workspaces. Natural light is far better for people than fluorescent lighting. Simply introducing plants into an office environment improves physical and mental health.

1% TIP: RETHINK YOUR OFFICE SPACE

In the last decade, there have been great advances in how companies use workspaces to inspire excellent work. Ask yourself if the space that you, your coworkers, or your employees work in is set up to ensure optimal productivity and wellness. Simple changes such as modular furniture, quiet spaces, and improved natural lighting can have a significant effect on productivity. And whenever possible, think about getting away from your desk for an energizing change of scene.

The old standard environment, which consisted of little more than a desk, a chair, and a phone, is just not helping people do their best work anymore. Company leaders always need to consider if they are providing people with opportunities to be their best selves. Can they perform? Can they concentrate? Can they focus? Can they excel? Can they activate their brains? Can they improve their energy? Creating an environment where all these things are possible can make an enormous impact. Over the last ten to fifteen years, a lot of offices have been switched over to an open concept. The thought was it allowed people to work easier together and created fewer barriers by eliminating distinctions of who had an office and who didn't. At the same time, it also created an atmosphere where we don't have the ability to get deep into a task because you constantly risk being interrupted. People don't have the ability to be uninterrupted for extended periods. Again, this is why it's helpful to have private rooms where employees can make calls, conduct meetings, or simply take advantage of some quiet if need be.

We need to make sure that whatever we are trying to accomplish, the environment reflects that. For example, if you must be on a phone call, then go into an office or a boardroom and close the door so you're not disrupting everybody else around you. If you have to do some collaborative work, then get into a space where you can throw things up on the wall and be engaged with the people around you. I love meeting in places where people are encouraged to be engaged. When people can jot down thoughts on colorful Post-its and stick them to whiteboards, the creativity flows. If you are in an open concept office and you are finding it hard to focus, try to eliminate the distractions.

Noise-canceling headphones can help. They let others

around know you are working while helping you immerse yourself in your task. It's all about engineering your environment and using the power of ergonomics to make sure you can get your very best work done in the easiest possible way. It's also time for companies to realize people like to listen to music while working. It can actually be helpful to their productivity. Some people, such as myself, enjoy things like "Bright Minds: Memory Rescue Music" by Barry Goldstein and Daniel G. Amen to heighten focus and mental sharpness. Either way, discouraging headphone use is an antiquated practice.

1% TIP: USE HEADPHONES TO INCREASE PRODUCTIVITY

Gone are the days when wearing headphones or earbuds while working was viewed as a distraction. Whether it is at work, home, or on the road, having access to music or mindfulness audio that can assist with productivity is a way to ensure your work is optimally efficient.

I also encourage you to create a home office space that replicates some of these elements. With the growing opportunity for more and more people to work from home, it's crucial to have an environment that inspires you to do amazing work. I have set myself up at home in a space with artwork and a view. I can go into my home office, listen to music, and disconnect from the outside world in order to do my best work. If you are a person who frequently works remotely, it can help to also have a road warrior kit you can take on the road. Equip yourself with high-quality headphones, perhaps a journal or other meditation device—anything you need to create an environment where you can focus fully on your tasks.

THE COST OF DISTRACTION

Distractions are everywhere, especially in work environments where employees are doing the bulk of their jobs seated in front of computer screens. Just think about what you see when you walk around your own place of business. You see people reading nonwork-related articles online or scanning social media. You see them checking personal email accounts or visiting sites for their favorite stores to check out the deals of the day. You'll see them working as well, but these distractions are often too much for them to resist when they have constant internet access.

A Virgin Pulse study[12] shows 52 percent of respondents reported being distracted between 1 and 20 percent of the time while at work. Forty-three percent say they get distracted 21 to 75 percent of the time. Only 5 percent indicate they are constantly focused while at work.

---

12 "Driven by Distractions: Why Employees' Focus Is Waning at Work & What You Can Do about It," *Virgin Pulse*, October 22, 2014, https://www.virginpulse.com/press/95-of-employees-are-distracted-during-the-workday-new-virgin-pulse-survey-finds/.

Common sources of digital distraction include:

- checking texts
- checking emails
- online shopping
- social media
- reading blogs
- checking news sites
- planning vacations online
- paying bills online

Technology is not the only thing to blame. Other factors employees commonly waste time on are:

- socializing with colleagues
- unnecessary meetings
- personal phone conversations
- micromanagement
- visiting the kitchen, water cooler, or break room

1% TIP: ELIMINATE DISTRACTIONS

Spend some time making a list of all the things that distract you from your work during a typical workday such as email, social media, socializing, or surfing websites. From there, commit to a plan that will eliminate these distractions during work time so that you can amplify your productivity.

Here are some more interesting numbers to consider:

- Three minutes—How frequently the average office worker is interrupted or distracted, according to the University of California, Irvine
- Twenty-three minutes—How long it takes to return to a task after being interrupted, according to the University of California, Irvine
- Eight—Average number of windows open on a worker's computer at the same time, according to *The Overflowing Brain: Information Overload and the Limits of Working Memory* by Torkel Klingberg
- Thirty—Average number of times per hour an office worker checks their email inbox, according to the National Center for Biotechnology Information[13]

For many companies, all this wasted time results in significant financial losses. According to research published by Basex, a knowledge economy research firm, information overload cost the US economy at least $997 billion per year in reduced productivity and innovation as of 2010.[14]

To be fair, this age of constantly being connected is not just an employee issue. We as employers need to accept

---

13   "Neuroscience: The Next Competitive Advantage," *Think Better*, https://www.steelcase.com/research/articles/topics/open-plan-workplace/think-better/.

14   Jonathan B. Spira, "Information Overload Now $997 Billion: What Has Changed?" *Basex*, December 16, 2010, http://www.basexblog.com/2010/12/16/io-997/.

responsibility for our role in creating and perpetuating the problem. At what point over the last ten to fifteen years did it become acceptable for us as employers to send emails, texts, and information to our employees 24/7? I don't think it was totally intentional, but many employers think nothing of sending an employee an email in the evening or on the weekend. I used to be the worst. I travel a lot, and I would see time on a plane as extremely productive. I would often compose sixty to a hundred emails during a flight. When I landed and connected to hotel Wi-Fi, regardless of the time of day, this barrage of emails would hit cyberspace. I had somehow become unaware of the fact that one of our employees might well be out for dinner with their spouse (who isn't happy to begin with about how little time they have together) only to receive an email from the president on a company-paid phone, feeling an obligation to read, and possibly respond. Managers have to think about what might be happening in the employee's life when they hit Send. To managers, it's just another email, something to cross off the to-do list. To the employee, it's a complete disruption of whatever they were doing. Imagine being out to dinner with the family for a birthday celebration on a Saturday night and getting an email from the boss about a problem you'll need to address first thing Monday. Most likely, your mood, if not the whole evening, is now ruined. The truth is, managers have no right contacting an employee in the evening or on the weekend, unless it is an emergency, which—let's be honest—it never is.

The good news is, there is a fix. I encourage you to do what I have done at our head office and what I encourage all of my colleagues to do: set up an automatic notification policy on your servers that does not allow emails to be sent or received before 6:00 a.m., after 6:00 p.m., or on the weekend. Ours reads: "AMJ has developed a work-life balance program where we do not send or receive emails before 6:00 a.m., after 6:00 p.m., or on the weekend. If you are a valued customer who needs to reach me before then, please do not hesitate to reach me at _____, or our 24-hour customer service center at _____."

1% TIP: LIMIT EXPECTATIONS
FOR CHECKING EMAIL

Consider a company-wide commitment that eliminates the expectation to check emails between 6:00 p.m. and 6:00 a.m. the next day or on weekends. Publicize this policy on your servers and ensure that managers model the new guidelines for everyone else. Offer clients and staff a number to call if there is a legitimate emergency. Ensure managers respect the parameters when communicating with employees.

The truth is, there are very few occasions where something is urgent enough that it requires an immediate response. In the first six months that I had the autoresponse, I did not receive one urgent call—in fact, I received several responses from people praising us for putting such measures in place. Most companies that deal with time-sensitive or customer service issues have staff who are dedicated to managing phones or online chat channels. It doesn't mean that you or I can't work outside of those hours if we have things that must be done, but it does mean that the recipient doesn't have to have their dinner or weekend interrupted by something that can wait.

In the time before email and texting, which really wasn't that long ago, if I needed to reach someone in the evening or on the weekend, I had to pick up the phone and call them. The fact that I had to call them would cause me to think about whether they might be at dinner or enjoying their family on the weekend and I never called them. Today, we have become numb or oblivious to what the recipient of a communication might be doing when we hit Send.

We are already starting to see some countries introduce legislation that prohibits employers from communicating with employees outside of work hours. If we are not paying for 24/7, why should we expect it is all right to communicate 24/7?

Many employees have become fatigued with the sense that they don't have evenings and weekends to themselves. It is ruining relationships, causing burnouts and anxiety, and creating an unsustainable pace for employees. I don't think most of us as employers even set out to think that we would one day have 24/7 access to our employees—we simply got lulled into it. If as an employer the idea of shutting down email between certain hours every day seems too big a step, try doing it just on the weekends.

I thought that when we first implemented our email policy that there would be an outcry, but the response from peers, customers, and employees has been a resounding, "Great idea. We should be doing this." In fact, in all the time since we started doing this, I have never once had anyone field a complaint because they weren't immediately reachable.

I started this section by saying that an employee head count has increased over the last ten years at a far faster rate than our revenues, and it is because we are seeing a decline in productivity related to employees being distracted more than 30 percent of their day. Many other companies have experienced the same phenomenon, and it all links back to productivity. It is no coincidence these trends coincide with the rise of smartphones and other technology. These things that are supposed to make us function at a higher level are also capable of stealing our attention and making us less productive.

If we are productive only 70 percent of the time, the reason so many companies are suffering is not a guessing game; it's a simple math equation. They are losing money both from an operational standpoint as well as from the drain on employee benefits all this distraction causes. Stressed-out employees are often unhealthier employees. They use more sick days and experience frequent burnout, all of which impacts the bottom line. More importantly, it impacts their overall well-being.

THE SOLUTION IS FOCUS

When business leaders understand how distraction affects the workforce, they can make changes to improve everything from overall employee satisfaction to the company's bottom line. Management of California-based Tower Paddle Boards realized this and attacked the problem with a creative and effective solution. (Much of the following information comes from "What Happened When I Moved My Company to a 5-Hour Workday," an October 30, 2016, article by Stephan Aarstol for www.fastcompany.com.)

Founders of the business created it based on their love of paddle boarding. But once profits starting soaring, no one at the company had any time for their favorite hobby anymore. Everyone was too busy working. They needed a change.

To give employees their lives back, company founder Stephan Aarstol implemented a five-hour workday. Everyone started work at 8:00 a.m., and as long as they proved to be highly productive, they were permitted to leave at 1:00 p.m.

Aarstol also offered monetary incentive for his employees' heightened focus. He rolled out a 5 percent profit sharing at the same time. Now, someone making $40,000 a year stood to make $8,000 more, all while working 750 fewer hours. It didn't cost the company a single dime. There was no financial risk to the bottom line.

All he asked for in exchange was that each team member be twice as productive as they had been previously. He set the bar high, and his employees met the challenge. Their work week became better than most people's vacation weeks.

Financially, the results were astounding. They were listed in *Inc.* 5000 list of America's fastest-growing companies two years in a row. They had a ten-person team that generated $9 million in revenues. In the first year of the changes, their annual revenues were up 40 percent.

> **1% TIP: EXCHANGE TIME FOR PRODUCTIVITY**
>
> Engage your employees in a conversation about making work time much more effective so that you can all enjoy a better work-life balance. Working together to monitor the overall effectiveness of everything from meetings to email communications or individual work can enable a widespread improvement in overall effectiveness and a simultaneous improvement in joy and wellness.

Tower is just one example of how better focus means

greater satisfaction, both in our personal lives and in our work environments. Most business professionals waste the bulk of their day on unnecessary distractions. The average worker receives 109 emails a day.[15] The barrage of distractions is incessant, and each one pulls focus from the task at hand. Taking control of how we use our time and energy allows us to become less wasteful and more productive, and the first step in doing so is to focus.

Imagine a Major League Baseball playoff game. It's the bottom of the ninth, and the game is on the line. For both the pitcher and the hitter, this is a career- and life-defining moment. The crowd is going crazy. Tension is soaring. The two are completely focused on each other, until the pitcher looks up into the stands. In that moment, he's lost his focus and will likely not be able to perform, at least not at the level he usually does. Yet in our own lives, we expect to be able to perform at our best when distracted all the time. We sit at our desks attempting to work until we get an email or our social media post gets a new like. It is like we are the pitcher and all those distractions are the rowdy crowd.

Getting focused requires simply putting specific strategies, tools, and tactics in place, then building new habits. We

---

15 Joe Robinson, "There Are Always a Million Distractions. Here's How to Silence the Noise and Pay Attention," *Entrepreneur*, September 2014, https://www.entrepreneur.com/article/236395#.

must relearn how to direct our attention in the face of distraction. This is a fundamental skill all athletes learn. It is why a pitcher in a baseball game can tune out the crowd. It enables Olympic athletes to forget the fact they are being watched by millions of viewers. It is an essential skill in the world of competitive sports, and there are simple ways we can apply it to our own lives.

TOOLS AND TACTICS FOR FOCUS

Focus is not just important for our health and well-being; it can help protect our futures. In this day of artificial intelligence and other technology replacing humans in many workforce roles, we must stay competitive. We can do so by constantly developing our ability to be creative and maintaining our problem-solving skills.

Being responsive rather than reactive is critical. We are living through the biggest revolution in the way we work since our economy transitioned from agricultural to industrial a hundred years ago. We're now transitioning from industrial to technological.

Many industries are being disrupted. In the world of finance, automated investing with algorithms that beat 95 percent of investment professionals are leading entire generations to put their money into companies such as Wealthsimple and Wealthfront. As a result, traditional investing firms are being squeezed out, because they can't beat the computer.

Artificial intelligence even affects the way we get around. Every day, we move closer to automated cars becoming the norm. The car industry is one of the top employers for most of North America. As the technology evolves, many people will be out of a job.

We, as humans, need to adapt to this new landscape. We need to be able to provide experiences and be agile in our thinking. We must provide better products, better services, and more value to our clients. We need to be able to think up new things. We need to be able to create new ideas. Problem solving, creativity, and agile thinking is the future. It's essential. If you are not capable of that, you have no hope for the future. You're simply going to be railroaded by what's coming.

To possess any of these qualities, you must first have the ability to focus. You need to be able to work without distraction, create an environment where you can be creative, and build routines that activate your brain and help you learn better.

Because of this, we also need a new way of working. Successful companies are understanding this more and more and creating workspaces conducive to such practices.

These companies are attracting and retaining some of the world's top talent. We will delve deeper into the specific tools needed for improved focus in chapter 12.

THE VALUE OF PRESENTISM

Everything outlined in this book thus far is about constructing a workday where you are exponentially healthier and higher performing at the same time. Perhaps even more importantly, it can allow you to increase your presentism.

Presentism is the opposite of absenteeism. It is when your mind and body are both engaged in the same activity. It might sound simple, but it does not come easily for most people. How many times have you been physically at work but mentally at home? Your body is at your desk, but your brain is focused on something you're worried about, maybe a broken appliance or an upcoming doctor's appointment or an argument with your children or spouse. You're super stressed because of something that's happening, just can't let it go, and your mind is not in a great place.

You are incapable of producing your best work when you are in such a state. Focus, achieved by way of all the examples set forth in previous chapters, allows you to be in the present, where only what's immediately in front of you controls your attention.

From an employer standpoint, presentism means money. In my work with organizations where we've implemented programs aimed at improving health, well-being, and human performance, I've seen a 1.8:1 return on investment for every $1 spent. For every dollar invested in improving health and well-being in the workplace, you are making even more. Far beyond that, you are seeing happier, healthier, more engaged employees who like coming to work and who stick around longer.

CHAPTER 8

The Focused Culture

As we have said previously, it's time to stop thinking of work as a marathon and start thinking of it as a series of sprints. When you approach work with great energy and deep focus and allow yourself time to recover and regenerate, you can truly hone in on what matters most.

We want to create a happier, healthier world by changing how we work. The grind of the Cult of Busyness drains us of our energy and takes a toll on our well-being. We must stop living this way if we ever want to truly maximize our potential and reach our goals.

Years ago, the thinking around athletes training for the Olympics (really, all professional athletes) was, "Go as hard as you can as often as you can." It was all about putting in the most volume possible. Whoever didn't get sick or injured made the Olympic team.

This approach led to very short careers. Most athletes stopped competing in their late teens or early twenties. This went on until the early 1990s, when a cultural shift happened in coaching that completely revolutionized the field. Athletes still trained at a very high level, but training was interspersed with more recovery time. They started incorporating nutrition, massage, and sleep into their routines to help them recover and regenerate faster.

This is the same approach we need to adopt in business. We need to think about it in terms of our ability to work at a high level and then recover and regenerate so we can end up healthier, higher performing, and ultimately, happier. Work should not be a sixty-plus-hour task seen as nothing more than drudgery. All great employers should truly want their employees to live fulfilling lives, not waste away on the path to burnout.

WHAT EMPLOYEES WANT

Over the last ten years, some of the brightest minds coming out of the younger generations have been drawn to companies that focus on lifestyle and balance. This generation has no interest in the traditional highly structured, "work until you drop" eight-hour workday. They want a flexible work schedule and more balance in their lives.

When I was beginning my employment, the mindset was

that whoever got to the office first and left last got noticed. There were countless times when I dragged my body into the office early in the morning so I could be there before everybody else, and I'd wait until the last person left so I could leave after them. I thought this automatically meant I was being productive. It didn't. It just meant I was doing something arbitrary so I could be recognized.

The old cliché "The early bird gets the worm" is no longer true. It's been replaced with "The second mouse gets the cheese." We all know what happens to the first mouse—it gets trapped. This is exactly what's happening with the workplace today. People looking for work are not interested in getting into the grind they saw their parents live. It doesn't mean they're not prepared to work. They are just working smarter.

Attracting and retaining great employees requires some radical thinking around the way we've done things. Shorter workdays are a great place to start. Allowing employees to work fewer hours shows you value the lifestyle-workplace balance. It sends the message of, *Yes, we expect you to work well, and we're going to teach you how to be more productive, and we're going to provide you with the right tools to be focused, but we're not going to bug you in the evenings. We're not going to bug you on the weekends. You can have a highly productive career working six, seven, or eight hours a day. You can be more present and engaged outside of work hours.*

Many of the most successful corporations of the last decade are doing this already. They offer more flexibility. They have built health, lifestyle, and balance directly into their programs. The Googles, Facebooks, Apples, and other new tech companies are reaping the benefits of implementing these practices. They also are attracting top talent. They must be doing something right.

WHAT EMPLOYERS WANT

Shorter days aren't just good for the employee. They're good for the whole company, as reducing unproductive hours will improve your bottom line and reduce costs.

There's going to be a reduction in benefits used. When we made these changes at our company, we saw sick days decrease significantly. It makes sense because employees are healthier, less stressed, eating better, and better educated about how to care for themselves and maintain a lifestyle-work balance. You'll also notice people actually want to come to work because they look forward to being more productive.

Because employees are happier, they will stay in their jobs longer. You're going to have less turnover, so you will save on the astronomical costs of hiring and training new employees. Focused employees increase their productivity and get more done in less time—employers should want that.

Finally, they are wasting less time, so you are wasting less money. If the average employer believes his employees are spending 30 to 50 percent of their workday distracted, why wouldn't he want to change that?

LEADING BY EXAMPLE

In places of business, there are ways management can help employees find flow. A 2014 *Business Insider* article[16] explains why LinkedIn's CEO Jeff Weiner devoted thirty- to ninety-minute time slots each day for personal time, coaching, and reflection. Weiner said he started using this approach when he realized his schedule was so full of back-to-back meetings that he had no time to think.

The article reports he first felt like this unstructured time was an indulgence but soon realized it was vital to his job performance. He spent the time "getting to know his team and coaching them to solve problems on their own (rather than just telling them what to do, which seems easier, but would actually cost him more time in the long run); strategic thinking; and reflecting on his company's mission."

To allow his staff to have similar experiences, Weiner also required his leadership team have no meetings, phone

---

16 Jacquelyn Smith, "Why LinkedIn's CEO Jeff Weiner Schedules Blocks of 'Nothing' into His Calendar," *Business Insider*, November 4, 2014, http://www.businessinsider.com/linkedins-jeff-weiner-schedules-blocks-of-nothing-2014-11.

calls, or distractions for the first two hours of their morning each day.

They were to spend the time focused on charting the strategic direction of the organization.

Not long after implementing the change, the company was sold to Microsoft. It is interesting that top people at one of the largest social networks in the world—who are supposed to be communicating and constantly engaged—understood the need to disconnect and focus to make real progress.

EMAIL POLICIES

There are many practices you can put in place to curb email distraction. To avoid the never-ending onslaught, you can batch your emails. Batching, a concept developed by Tim Ferriss, is setting aside a specific time to check emails and not allowing them to distract you otherwise. For example, you might set aside the last fifteen minutes of every hour to check emails. You might designate certain hours of the day when you check them. You turn off notifications and do not allow them to pull your attention away from the task at hand. There are many software programs that allow you to block email during certain times.

If you're not sure how much of your time email is stealing, track it. Start a journal to record how much time you actually spend on emails a day. Then take that time and break it into focused sections. Instead of spending two minutes here and thirty minutes there, set aside a specific ten or fifteen minutes at regular stages of the day to tackle them. Treat these sessions like sprints you do throughout the day.

I've been batching my communications twice a day. I'll do a quick scan in the morning just to look for anything interesting and then push it all off until 11:00 a.m. Then I'll do another batch at 4:00 p.m. If anything's urgent, I deal with it right away, but then I put it away because I know my best work is done from 8:00 a.m. to 11:00 a.m. I will focus in on my most important work, and then from 11:00 a.m. to noon, I'll try to hammer through as much email as I can, then turn it off again until 4:00 p.m., and then deal with whatever came through during the day. Instead of responding to things constantly all day long, I do it at very specific times. This practice allows me to enter into a focused state of flow, which is where I do my best work.

People think not checking emails constantly takes great discipline, but this is not the case. It definitely required some systematic processes to be put in place. I had to build a new habit to break the old one. I was connected constantly, and I would respond to anyone who emailed me almost instantly. I was known for that. My work allows me to have a global reach, so people all over the world are contacting me frequently. For a while, I was priding myself on the fact I would always respond to people, and they could count on my getting back to them. But then I came to the realization that this behavior is not necessarily a good thing.

In order to have an impact in the world, which is what I'm trying to do, you cannot constantly react to people's instantaneous communications. It costs too much time to move from task to task to task. It keeps me from doing my best work. Today, I have turned off all notifications on my phone, my Apple Watch, and my computer. I have the "do not disturb" on my computer all the time. I get no notifications, no buzzes, no pings, nothing.

Instead, I actually have communication time blocked in my schedule now, and my assistants never schedule during that time. I've become very deliberate about structuring my days in such a way that I'm doing my most important work when it matters to me the most.

Granted, this doesn't work for everybody. If someone is in sales or customer service and their important task needs to be responding to customers or clients, emails can't always be ignored. If that's your number one job, then that needs to be your priority. Figure out what other factor is distracting you, and eliminate it instead.

We also encourage employees to disengage from email outside of business hours. They can set up an automated reply message explaining that messages received after 6:00 p.m. or before 6:00 a.m. Monday to Friday and during the weekends will be responded to on the next business day. They can indicate that if the matter is urgent, contacting them on a cell is appropriate. The response has been resoundingly positive.

Another thing that evolved out of our project is a change to the way we write emails. We all know that we appreciate and respect one another. When we write emails, we don't need to begin by saying, "Hi, Bruce. I hope you had a good weekend. I hope the kids are well. I hope everything else is well." We don't waste people's time. Instead, we get right to the point. This is the part of texting I like. It forces you to be concise, reinforcing the lesson that less is more.

We also started using Slack, a communication tool that allows you to create channels, which are effectively projects, that include only the relevant people. When you do communicate using that venue, you don't use a subject button. You don't need to comb through a contacts list. Everyone will see whatever you post. It's almost like texting. It's short, quick, and very effective. Slack also allows us to block and save messages between 8:00 p.m. and 8:00 a.m. They won't notify us of the messages until the next morning. This frees everyone from feeling the need to be chained to their phones or computers during downtime.

We do not allow arguing in emails. People are more inclined when using email to say things they would not say to someone in person, and you can't take back what's been written. If you have an issue that has potential to become an argument, it's smarter to think carefully about what you want to say, then pick up the phone.

We also discourage copying everyone on everything. There used to be a day when anytime our managers did anything good, I got copied on it. Anytime something bad happens, I get copied on it. It was driving me crazy because they never stopped. During one of our regular conference calls, I said to the team, "Folks, I know you do a great job. Let's have a bragging session once every six months where we talk about the wonderful things we're doing, but please don't send me an email or copy me on an email because it clutters my box. Definitely don't tell me about all the problems we're having unless you need my involvement in solving them." I went from being copied a hundred times a day to ten.

Finally, consider using the phone. In this digital age, we tend to see talking on the phone as an outdated practice, but there are times when it can be far more efficient than email, particularly if the topic requires a lot of back and forth. If you have an issue that would be better handled on the phone, schedule time to call the people to talk them through it. It will save everyone time in the long run.

1% TIP: AUDIT YOUR COMMUNICATION PRACTICES

Are there ways to improve your individual or collective communication? Can you use a platform such as Slack to centralize messages? Could emails be more succinct? Can you reduce needless CCs? Are there times when a call would be easier than another email?

AVOID UNNECESSARY MEETINGS

Everyone dislikes meeting for the sake of meeting. Regular management and staff meetings can be a waste of people's time. Meetings should be very specific. They should have a detailed agenda, a start, and a finish. They should include only people who absolutely must be there. And there's no reason meetings must last the standard thirty or sixty minutes. Make them five or ten minutes if that's all the time you really need. You'll find you can save a lot of time in meetings if you set the expectation that they will not include an initial ten minutes of small talk. Don't waste people's time with catching up and idle chat—save that for the break room. If you are in a meeting that's been scheduled for thirty minutes and it ends early, don't force everyone to stay and waste that time. Instead, use it to do something healthy, such as taking a walk. Finally, push more meetings to the phone rather than forcing everyone to gather in person. I find it moves things along faster and cuts out much of the wasted time. If you are meeting in person, however, phones should be off. The less potential for distraction, the less potential for wasted time.

Personally, I see meetings as the bane of my existence. I do everything in my power to avoid them at all cost. When they're essential, they're essential. But the vast majority of the time, they're a complete waste. I take many steps to ensure meetings are as short as they possibly can be.

Meetings that bring people together to create things or to solve problems are wonderful, but the traditional meetings that are only about updates and sharing information put me to sleep. Just like any other distraction, do not let them hinder your focus.

DEVICE-FREE WORK TIME

You can begin to show your team how effective they can be without distractions simply by banning phones from meetings or group work scenarios. When we have our think tank sessions or board meetings, we ask people to shut down their phones. We have a basket they can leave them in, or they can leave them with our receptionist who can keep an eye on them in case of emergency. It adds structure to your meetings to acknowledge *we are going to be more productive if we're not on our phones.*

Nothing is more frustrating than to see people texting while somebody is speaking on a point. What message are we sending people when we do this? We know we can't do two things at the same time effectively, so when you are on your phone, you are telling somebody you're not interested in what they are saying. Besides such behavior being extremely rude, it's sending the very clear message that we simply don't care enough to give them our full attention.

This also puts the responsibility on the person running the meetings to be efficient and effective and to not waste anyone's time. If the meeting is being run effectively and decisions are being made and input is being given, it becomes a lot easier to put away your cell phone. You should be completely engaged.

It's all about focus with the added element of time responsibility. We all must make sure we are using everyone's time effectively.

COMMUNICATION IS KEY

When implementing change, clear communication is crucial. If people are confused, they don't do it. If there is the slightest shred of doubt in the employee's mind about whether something is OK or expected, change will not happen.

Talk to employees often about the benefits of these changes so they understand fully how they will improve many aspects of their lives both at and outside of work. We sent out weekly emails with information about the benefits of focus and concentration, which employees really enjoyed. People printed them off and saved them for future use. You could hold lunch-and-learn sessions, write about it in your company newsletter, or find your own creative way to communicate to the team.

Show them examples of how new companies are working, such as Amazon, Uber, Facebook, and Google. These multimillion-dollar companies are the future and are growing because they are attracting the best talent in the world. They all operate with these new strategies already in place, and because of it, people want to work there.

Millennials especially want balance in their lives. They are not drawn to workplaces that demand 24/7 access and long hours. They are not even solely concerned about money. They want a company that can offer them a certain lifestyle.

The most successful companies are thinking about the overall health of the employee. They are not trying to wring every last ounce of energy out of everybody but enabling employees to think, be creative, problem solve, be agile, come up with solutions to difficult problems, or just get the job done so they can leave and recover, regenerate, have a life, and be part of the organization for many years to come. The millennial generation has less loyalty to companies, so the likelihood of their moving around to get more experiences is higher. It behooves us to try and create better environments for people so we can retain our talent.

WALK THE WALK

Many company leaders have benefits that include health care and annual exams, but I'm continuously shocked by the number of CEOs who are out of shape physically and who have no sort of balance in their work and personal lives. I've gone to lunch with folks who would order a burger and fries every time. To me, that's a surefire way to guarantee you'll need a nap in the afternoon. It begs the question, how effective are these people really?

We've had a bit of this Hollywood/rock star CEO syndrome over the last ten to fifteen years where the CEOs act more like movie stars than true leaders. That attitude can be a difficult thing for a board to address. The last thing you want to do is tell someone in authority that he or she needs to lose some weight, but it is up to a board governance committee to address the health issue of their CEO, just as they would the way he or she conducts themselves publicly and when representing the company.

We are seeing a bit of a shift where now the good health and the fitness of the CEO is almost expected. We call it the "corporate Olympian" or the "corporate athlete" concept. People are beginning to understand that to a certain degree, it reflects on the ability of the individual to execute, to be able to travel well, to be able to handle stress, and to have the energy that you would expect to be able to serve the company.

Leaders can also serve as an example by working reasonable hours. If the employer is the one coming in working sixty to seventy hours a week, no employee is ever going to feel OK cutting back their own hours. Many times in my career, I've brought an employee in who is working way too many hours and I said to him, "Look, if you're working more than forty hours a week, we need to hire a second person, take away some of your responsibilities, or find ways to make you more efficient. But at the end of the day, I do not want you consistently working more than forty hours a week." It's important to stress to employees that it's the long game that matters. People work grueling hours thinking they will one day be "caught up." The truth is, there will always be more work to do. That does not mean, however, that you cannot disconnect from work and shut it down when appropriate. Remember, always having something to do is a good thing. It's why you have a job.

Employers should coach their employees to find ways to create balance in their lifestyle. Let them know working that much is not what we want as a company or what you want as a leader. Tell them, "If you're trying to impress me, you're not doing it. I will be more impressed when you manage your work to the point where you are able to go home."

Leaders set the pace by their willingness to walk the walk. If leaders are eating well, looking after themselves, and limiting emails, employees will feel more motivated to do the same. I was once on holiday when I received an email from one of my employees, a second request regarding a non-urgent issue. I sent him a note back explaining the reason he wasn't getting a response was because I was on vacation. In so many words, I told him to drop it. Sometimes you have to be blunt to get people to understand.

I have seen leaders say, "Oh yeah, I think it's important that everybody works out. I think it's important for people to eat better. I think it's important for people to get lots of sleep," and yet they're not working out when they are at work, their food is not optimal, and they are exhausted and stressed. Unless they actually practice what they preach, employees won't buy it. They need to see the leader putting on his shoes to go out for a walk. They need to see him eating a healthy lunch. Walking the walk publicly is key.

For change to stick, you need management to buy into it and to be on the same page as the employees so they can feel extremely comfortable following new strategies. If management tells employees they're not expected to be working on evenings and weekends, management can't be working on evenings and weekends. Walking the walk conveys the message that you actually care about your employees and want them to be happy. You have to lead this cultural change.

Work Mastery Checklist

OVERVIEW

North American work culture is full of habits, tendencies, and assumptions about how we work. Many of these biases and beliefs are counterproductive and undermine the effectiveness and well-being of individuals and teams. They also have a big negative impact on the bottom line. Employees, employers, and organizations that understand the Focus Effect and adopt an approach that reflects an understanding of the conditions for optimal work and wellness are setting themselves apart.

THE QUIZ

Answer the questions below to assess how well your work

and work environment are set up to generate optimal focus, wellness, and productivity. Your responses will assist you in identifying simple changes you can make to get more out of your time, enjoy your life and work, and elevate your performance individually and as a group.

DIRECTIONS

Select the answer that best matches your current situation. Your responses will give you a sense of how you are supporting your ability to achieve the Focus Effect. Add up your scores at the end to see how you are doing. You can then make minor changes by addressing one question at a time. Then come back in a couple of months to take the quiz again and see how your focus has improved!

1. DO YOU AVOID MULTITASKING?

- Always (5 points)
- Yup (4 points)
- Pretty much (3 points)
- Sort of (2 points)
- Not really (1 point)
- Never (0 points)

Recommendations: When you are working on a task, do it and it alone until it is complete, without allowing your attention to be diverted to anything else.

Rationale: Our brains are truly not capable of multitasking. We cannot do two things at once. We might think we are tackling more than one activity simultaneously when in reality, all we are doing is switching back and forth from one task to another. Every time we switch, we lose focus and have to reorient our brains, and that does not happen as quickly as we think. Research shows it takes an average of fifteen minutes to reorient yourself to a primary task after a distraction, which results in a 40 percent drop in productivity.[17] Not to mention that multitasking hurts cognitive performance and short-term memory and can temporarily reduce IQ by fifteen points.[18]

2. DO YOU PUT YOUR DEVICE ON "DO NOT DISTURB" DURING MEETINGS AND TASKS?

- Always (5 points)
- Yup (4 points)
- Pretty much (3 points)
- Sort of (2 points)
- Not really (1 point)
- Never (0 points)

Recommendations: While working on a project or attending a meeting, having a conversation or manag-

---

17 Atchley, "You Can't Multitask."

18 Alban, "The Cognitive Costs of Multitasking."

ing a task, shut down all incoming notifications that will demand your attention.

Rationale: Your brain is wired to scan the environment for novelty, changes, and threats. When you let a barrage of bings, buzzes, rings, and pops assault your senses, your brain will be constantly interrupted, reducing your effectiveness and elevating your state of agitation. By eliminating all distractions when it matters, the quality and efficiency of your work will increase while your stress declines. The reality is that whatever is coming in can most often be managed when you are finished.

3. DOES YOUR SPACE (AND HOW YOU USE IT) PROMOTE WELLNESS AND PRODUCTIVITY?

- Always (5 points)
- Yup (4 points)
- Pretty much (3 points)
- Sort of (2 points)
- Not really (1 point)
- Never (0 points)

Recommendations: Assess your workspace and how you interact with it to ensure you are applying best practices. For example, there are several ways to alter the physical environment to change the way you work, including standing, walking, or flexible desks; bar stools and high tables; chairs designed to move; walking meetings; off-site meetings; meditation rooms; vending machines with healthy food choices; and natural light.

Rationale: There is a significant link between space, furniture and equipment, and our effectiveness and well-being. Companies that utilize advanced thinking about the environment in which their employees work have found high levels of wellness, productivity, efficiency, creativity, and overall performance.

4. DO YOU MONITOR AND LIMIT DISTRACTIONS?

- Always (5 points)
- Yup (4 points)
- Pretty much (3 points)
- Sort of (2 points)
- Not really (1 point)
- Never (0 points)

Recommendations: Conduct an assessment of the various distractions that interrupt you during the workday. Consider the range of technological distractions such as checking texts or emails, shopping online, social media, blogs and news sites, and paying bills online. Also, look at ways that you inadvertently waste time during the workday, such as socializing with colleagues, unnecessary meetings, personal phone conversations, micromanagement, and visiting the kitchen, water cooler, or break room. Once you have a clear sense of the ways that you are getting distracted from optimal work, make a plan to have a distinct line between when you are working and when you are taking a break or recreating. By stopping these behaviors, you will take control of your workflow and radically improve your focus.

Rationale: Studies show the average employee in 2016 spends 30–50 percent of his or her day digitally distracted. A Virgin Pulse study[19] shows 52 percent of respondents reported being distracted between 1 and 20 percent of the time while at work. Forty-three percent say they get distracted 21–75 percent of the time. Only 5 percent indicate they are constantly focused while at work. When we are unaware of the sources of distraction and their impact on our work, there is very little we can do about it. When we address the sources of distraction, we are happier, more productive, and more effective.

5. DO YOU HAVE A COMPANY POLICY THAT LIMITS TIMES FOR EMAIL RESPONSES?

- Always (5 points)
- Yup (4 points)
- Pretty much (3 points)
- Sort of (2 points)

---

19   "Driven by Distractions," *Virgin Pulse.*

- Not really (1 point)
- Never (0 points)

Recommendations: Set up an automatic notification policy on your servers that does not allow emails to be sent or received before 6:00 a.m., after 6:00 p.m., or on the weekend.

Rationale: At heart, every employee wants to do a good job. When an email comes in, whether it is from a boss, coworker, client, or supplier, there is immediate pressure for a person to reply, which creates perpetual anxiety and keeps people from genuinely relaxing at home so they are recovered and ready to excel when they get back to work. The problem is that it takes gravitas for an individual to set limits on their email use if those around them aren't doing so as well. By making it company policy, you protect everyone's time, and you set the entire organization up for optimal focus, impact, and well-being.

6. DO YOU FIND WAYS TO WORK BETTER IN LESS TIME?

- Always (5 points)
- Yup (4 points)
- Pretty much (3 points)
- Sort of (2 points)
- Not really (1 point)
- Never (0 points)

Recommendations: Offer employees an opportunity to work shorter hours if they are more productive during the time they are at work, and the results will shock you. The quality of work will increase, performance will improve, and everyone will enjoy working. Meanwhile, employees will have more time to genuinely recover before returning to go hard again the next day.

Rationale: Habitual attitudes toward work are just that—habits. They have become ingrained in our culture and in our workplaces. By shifting people's emphasis from a passive sense that they work a certain amount each day no matter what to an active sense that they have control over the length of their workday and level of productivity, you can transform the baseline approach in your organization.

7. DO YOU ALTERNATE PERIODS OF INTENSE WORK WITH DELIBERATE BREAKS TO RECOVER?

- Always (5 points)
- Yup (4 points)
- Pretty much (3 points)
- Sort of (2 points)
- Not really (1 point)
- Never (0 points)

Recommendations: Rather than just grinding it out all day long and inevitably becoming taxed, distracted, and bored, adopt the approach that has become the norm for elite athletes. Remove all distractions and work intensely for ninety minutes. Then take a thirty-minute break to let your mind rest, restore your body through motion and nutritious fuel, and get away from your desk. Then come back and go for it again.

Rationale: The human brain can focus for only ninety minutes at a time before it needs a substantial break to restore blood glucose and oxygen. Grinding it out for longer than that is unrealistic and typically requires the stimulation of caffeine, sugar, or simple carbohydrates that will ultimately erode focus and well-being, even as it provides a temporary lift.

8. DO YOU BLOCK OFF TIME WHEN YOU ARE UNAVAILABLE?

- Always (5 points)
- Yup (4 points)
- Pretty much (3 points)
- Sort of (2 points)
- Not really (1 point)
- Never (0 points)

Recommendations: Apply the principles of Power Work by identifying the time of the day when you are most productive and blocking that time into your schedule as a period when you are not to be disturbed so you can concentrate exclusively on what matters the most.

Rationale: We all have times in the day when we are at our best. If we allow this precious time to be eaten up by minor interruptions and tasks that don't require major focus, we are wasting an opportunity to do a great job. Save the simpler tasks and low-energy activities for parts of the day when you are at a lower ebb, and use your Power Work time for whatever is the most important thing on your list. It's also important to consider making this company policy so that everyone is approaching their work with the same mindset and you can all support one another.

9. DO YOU BATCH YOUR EMAIL SESSIONS?

- Always (5 points)
- Yup (4 points)
- Pretty much (3 points)
- Sort of (2 points)
- Not really (1 point)
- Never (0 points)

Recommendations: Identify two or three times during the day when you will focus exclusively on your email and only manage it during those blocks of time. Also, let everyone you work with know that's how you approach it so they know when to expect a response.

Rationale: While it seems that a quick peek at your email does no harm, the reality is that as soon as you scan it, your brain goes to work on whatever is there. Not to mention that if you think you should be checking it all the time, you are in a state of constant low-level anxiety about what is waiting for you or about to come in. You can remove all of this by having a clear delineation of time for checking and replying to emails that will free you up to focus on the task at hand. And when you are checking email, you will be highly efficient with it because it is your sole focus. Obviously, if you are in a job that is more heavily focused on communication, your batches of email will occur more frequently, but the premise is the same. Do email when you are doing email, and don't do email when you are not. Your brain will thank you.

10. DO YOU AUDIT YOUR COMMUNICATION PRACTICES?

- Always (5 points)
- Yup (4 points)
- Pretty much (3 points)
- Sort of (2 points)
- Not really (1 point)
- Never (0 points)

Recommendations: Make a comprehensive and brutally honest assessment of all of your communication methods: meetings, calls, texts, email, conversations, and so on.

Where could it be more efficient and focused? How can you make changes that will improve your work individually and collectively? How can you cut down on wasted time and ineffective interactions? Are there platforms such as Slack that would enable more effective communication? Figure out what is off the mark and make a change.

Rationale: Communication is one of the most important components of work. By asking yourself how you can do it better—and working with those around you to make a shared commitment to a change—you can create a culture of focus.

11. DO YOU AVOID WASTEFUL MEETINGS?

- Always (5 points)
- Yup (4 points)
- Pretty much (3 points)
- Sort of (2 points)
- Not really (1 point)
- Never (0 points)

Recommendations: Assess the quality and efficiency of your meetings—in person and on conference calls—and identify ways that they can be as productive as possible. And always ask yourself if a meeting is really required or whether a phone call could suffice, or a handful of people could handle it rather than requiring a large group. Make meetings specific, have a detailed agenda, include only the people who absolutely have to be there, keep gatherings as short as possible, and avoid wasting time on small talk. And whenever you do meet, make it a device-free interaction so everyone is laser focused on the topic.

Rationale: Meetings are one of the biggest time wasters in any organization because there are so many ways they can become unproductive. Do whatever you can to change that—from hiring a consultant to help you design meetings that work to only meeting when it is absolutely necessary.

12. AS A LEADER, DO YOU WALK THE WALK?

- Always (5 points)
- Yup (4 points)
- Pretty much (3 points)
- Sort of (2 points)
- Not really (1 point)
- Never (0 points)

Recommendations: When your organization starts to explore ways to create a more focused, productive, and healthy culture, the widespread commitment to making a change has to be evident in the ongoing behavior of the leadership team. Implementation of suggestions to make teams more effective will only be possible with leadership buy-in. This applies to healthy eating, taking breaks, blocking off time for work on the most important task, adopting new approaches to communication, and being focused at all times.

Rationale: Walking the walk means you believe that these changes will help the company excel. It also conveys the message that you care about your employees and want them to be happy. Cultural change can only happen if the leaders show the way.

TOTAL SCORE

40+ points:
You are living the dream! You have set up your life to optimize your focus and ensure you perform at your best most of the time at work.

20-39 points:
You are getting there. Keep tweaking your approach to find more areas for focus in your work life.

0-19 points:
You have made a start, but there is work to be done. Pick one item from the quiz above and work on it this week. After you have made some changes in that area, you can come back and focus on another area for improvement.

PART 3

Life Mastery

. . . .

There is no passion to be found in playing small—
in settling for a life that is less than the one you
are capable of living.
—NELSON MANDELA

CHAPTER 9

Focus in Action

Even visionaries need to be reminded of the power of focus occasionally.

Elon Musk, founder and CEO of Tesla, SpaceX, and Solar-City, was not at his best in 2008. He was going through an acrimonious divorce from a popular Beverly Hills blogger, who was using her site to disparage him. Tesla was in the middle of the financial meltdown affecting all car companies at the time. SpaceX had launched several rockets, all of which had blown up. Funds were drying up, and no one knew if any of his companies would survive.

A fourth SpaceX launch was on the horizon, and Musk knew it had to be a success. It was the only way he could save all of his companies, because it could lead to contracts with NASA. Musk put Tesla on autopilot and moved all his attention, focus, energy, and team to SpaceX.

They eliminated all distractions and put all their efforts and energies into one specific task. When the day of the launch finally came, its failure would mean their own.

The rocket went up, made it into orbit, and had a successful flight. Musk signed a contract with NASA, and SpaceX has grown ever since. Tesla has gone on to be the most valuable auto company in the world.

The key to navigating any moment of crisis is focus. Just as Musk used it to fuel his vision, you, too, can use it to propel yourself to new heights. But keep in mind, you don't have to be a Musk or a Jobs or a Buffett to make these changes. Anyone, at any level, can improve overall happiness and focus in the workplace.

TECHNOLOGY TRANCES

In this day when it has become acceptable for us all to go through life distracted by our cell phones, we are no longer fully engaged in the world around us. Pay attention when you are out in public—whether you're walking down the street, riding the bus, shopping, or eating in a restaurant—nearly everyone around you will be focused on their phones. This behavior, which just a short while ago would have seemed bizarre, is considered OK by today's standards. We all do it, regardless of the potential dangers it poses.

If I need to check a text or look for an email while I'm walking (which is very seldom), I move off to the side and get out of everyone's way. Not plowing into someone when you're walking and texting is the new manners, but bumping into someone is only a mild consequence of constant distraction. The number one cause of auto and pedestrian accidents is distraction. We also are seeing it as the cause of more and more concussions. Governments around the world are taking action against such senseless accidents with legislation prohibiting texting in many different scenarios, including, in Canada, while walking in crosswalks. We are risking our physical well-being for a device we never needed just a few short years ago.

We also risk harming our relationships when we overuse technology. In his January 2017 piece for the *Huffington Post* titled, "Why Smart Phones Are Driving Everyone Insane," Dr. Travis Bradberry analyzed the results of a study out of the University of Southern California's Marshall School of Business of 554 working professionals. The study found 86 percent of respondents think it's inappropriate to answer phone calls during meetings, and 84 percent think it's inappropriate to write texts or emails during meetings. Bradberry explains that inappropriate smartphone use shows a lack of respect, attention, listening, power, self-awareness, and social awareness.[20]

---

20   Travis Bradberry, "Why Smart Phones Are Driving Everyone Insane," *Huffington Post*, January 8, 2017, https://www.huffingtonpost.com/dr-travis-bradberry/why-smart-phones-are-driv_b_13979154.html.

The bottom line is, when you place higher importance on a device over the people in front of you, you devalue the interaction and damage the relationship.

IMPACT AT HOME

We also pay a price for constant distraction in our personal lives. Think about the average family at the dinner table. Chances are, both parents and kids are more fully focused on their phones than on one another. Live conversation is swapped for texts and tweets, and it's rare if anyone exchanges anything other than, "Pass the peas." Even when parents set aside specific time to spend with their kids, they are not capable of engaging fully. How many times have we all seen a mother or father pushing their child on a swing set with one hand and scrolling on their phone with the other? Parents are using iPads and tablets as babysitters for their children. Our children are not learning the art of conversation; they are learning from their parents that it is OK to be disengaged and not present. I worry about what this will look like for these children when they are adults.

All this distraction is impacting our ability to connect with our loved ones, which is truly one of the most important things in life. Yet we still seem to keep giving our distractions more and more of our time. A 2015 study of smartphone users showed participants used their phones a mean of eighty-five times each day and spent five hours each day using their smartphone.[21]

We're even terrified to disengage when we're away from work. Just the idea of vacation sends some people into a panic. They assume everything will fall apart in their absence, or worse, they will be replaced the second their chair gets cold, so they spend the entire vacation responding to emails and taking calls. Time away from work should be devoted to recovery and regeneration. It allows us to come back reenergized with an increased capacity for creativity and problem solving. Yet we refuse to allow ourselves this time away because of the stress we put on ourselves to stay busy. Seventy percent of deaths in the Western world are caused by stress-related illness.

We are much better people when we are healthy and focused. To achieve this, we need a radically different approach to the way we live our lives. For starters, I'd recommend employers find a way to encourage people to disconnect on vacations by making it mandatory they turn on away messages in their email when they're gone. This will allow people to feel like they are able to fully disconnect without the expectation to respond even in their absence.

---

21 S. Andrews, D. A. Ellis, H. Shaw, and L. Piwek, "Beyond Self-Report: Tools to Compare Estimated and Real-World Smartphone Use," *PLOS ONE* 10, no. 10: e0139004, https://doi.org/10.1371/journal.pone.0139004.

TECHNOLOGY IS NOT THE PROBLEM—WE ARE

For some of us, the constant need to check our phones is more than habit. It is an addiction we've never seen before, and it's creating a new kind of anxiety affecting people of all ages. There is a physiological response every time we check our phones. A release of dopamine occurs when we see a new notification or a new "like" on something we posted. FOMO, or fear of missing out, is real—the average internet user is now on social media and messaging services for over two hours per day.[22]

In a 2017 article, "Why We Can't Look Away from Our Screens," the *New York Times* interviewed social psychologist Adam Alter about his book, *Irresistible: The Rise of Addictive Technology and the Business of Keeping Us Hooked.* Alter told the *Times*, "These new gadgets turn out to be the perfect delivery devices for addictive media. If games and social media were once confined to our home computers, portable devices permit us to engage with them everywhere. Today, we're checking our social media constantly, which disrupts work and everyday life. We've become obsessed with how many 'likes' our Instagram photos are getting instead of where we are walking and whom we are talking to."[23]

---

22   Jason Mander, "Daily Time Spent on Social Networks Rises to Over 2 Hours," *Global Web Index*, May 16, 2017, https://blog.globalwebindex.net/chart-of-the-day/daily-time-spent-on-social-networks/.

23   Claudia Dreifus, "Why We Can't Look Away from Our Screens," *New York Times*, March 6, 2017, https://www.nytimes.com/2017/03/06/science/technology-addiction-irresistible-by-adam-alter.html.

Greg argues that everyone has experienced the feeling of digital addiction at some point. I have experienced it myself during a trip I took to Ecuador to go climb Chimborazo in 2015. We were out of cell range, but that didn't stop me from feeling the urge to check my phone. That feeling lasted for three days, but once it was over and I had essentially gone through the withdrawal, I started to feel amazing. My brain felt better. I was more creative, I could think, and I could engage with people better. Ten days later, we were coming back into Quito, the capital of Ecuador, when we reconnected to the network. When I could see all the messages downloading and the pings happening, I felt a little sick. The anxiety began to build instantaneously. It made me realize this was not something I wanted to have so much control over me.

To be clear, I am not saying technology is the root of all evil. I love technology. There are many benefits to carrying around all the world's knowledge in our pockets all day. If we have a question about anything, the answer is a few taps away. We can use it to do our jobs and boost our businesses. The danger comes when we use it constantly and are not able to disconnect. There are times during the day when we need to be separated from our devices. We need to put them down to exercise, spend time with our family, and be creative. Recognizing this and making a conscious decision to disengage can free us from becoming slaves to our devices.

The key to overcoming distraction addiction is deliberate focus. We need to find ways to control technology and not allow it to control us. Remember, technology is not the enemy. It can be part of the solution. There are computer programs that can help you block off notifications for designated lengths of time. You can set it up to remind you every few hours to check your social media devices. Doing this allows us to pull information in when we want it, rather than having it constantly pushed at us. It enables us to stop using technology blindly and become more purposeful with our behavior.

When we use focus to overcome our technology addiction, we become healthier and happier individuals and productive, more competitive employees.

WORDS OF WISDOM: DECATHLETE MIKE SMITH

A decathlon is ten separate sports within one competition, and therefore your focus is essential. You must put aside a previous event regardless of the outcome to focus on the next.

"The discipline is to let go of previous anchors, good or bad, and not as crucial to success," says Olympic decathlete Mike Smith.

So how do you do that? A key component of Smith's focus is acceptance. By accepting his performance, whether good or bad, he becomes almost like a third-party observer. Smith says he used to surrender to the extremes. But he soon learned to be able to move forward to perform well sometimes means giving something up.

We cannot be anchored in the past. We must be engaged in the present. If Smith is currently biking a challenging course, but his mind is back in the swimming competition, he is not allowing himself to perform to his full potential. In this race, his mind's involvement is as important as his body's.

In both his professional and personal life, Smith believes you must be able to let go and create space in your life for other positive things to enter. He is no stranger to overcoming negative experiences. In the 1996 Olympics, he was not performing the way he had hoped. He ended up experiencing what he describes as nonhysterical panic. He sought medical treatment but still felt himself spiraling downward.

With time, Smith was able to understand that while a failed Olympic performance can be devastating, it means little when compared to the importance of bigger things in life, such as family and friends. He got context. From that point on, he could look at his failures in the context of what really matters and move forward.

Smith has also enjoyed many successes. His fondest memory was of Götzis, the unofficial decathlon world championships. During the 1996 competition, Smith remembers being so focused that he almost felt like he was outside of his body. Throughout the competition, it was pouring down rain. Smith remained calm, focused, explosive, and energetic. He was totally in the zone, and he won the competition.

It wasn't until much later when he looked at the video of the events that he even realized it had been raining. He had been so deeply engaged in his task that he was completely oblivious to the horrific environmental conditions at the time. That's focus.

CHAPTER 10

The Focus Effect: Peak Performance

Part of the motivation behind the practices outlined in this book is to encourage industry leaders to change the culture of their existing businesses so they can be more attractive to young talent by offering a shorter workday, a more balanced lifestyle, and a healthier environment. In many ways, employers have allowed for the creation of the miserable workday epidemic—we must be the ones to swing the pendulum back. As leaders, we need to show people how these behaviors are harming their well-being and offer solutions for overcoming the problem.

We can learn from the examples of existing companies that are successfully incorporating this balance through the atmospheres they've created. These are some of the most successful companies of the last ten years. They're not just fun places to work; they're also attracting talent that's helping propel them to great heights. Businesses that remain reluctant to change must either accept second or third best when it comes to talent, or find ways to compete on a different playing field.

The success of our program lies in its ability to change the mindset of the employer to appreciate the employee more and allow them to do more in less time so they are free to have a healthier, more productive life outside the traditional nine-to-five. In the next chapter, we'll detail our specific approach to shorter workdays.

Many of us in business have followed the Googles and Amazons of the world at a glance, but we haven't peeled the covers back to see why they are still successful. Each one grew from the efforts of founders who did not like the traditional workspace and strove to do something different.

GOOGLE

The elements Google has put into place to create this type of a workplace are innovative and, as evidenced by their growth and success, highly effective. Nearly every aspect of their culture is linked to improving employee well-being and productivity.

A 2016 *Business Insider* article, "5 Reasons Google Is the

Best Place to Work in America and No Other Company Can Touch It," analyzes how the company topped *Business Insider*'s 2016 list of the fifty best companies to work for in America. The article shows:

- "Eighty-six percent of Google employees say they are either extremely satisfied or fairly satisfied with their job. More than 64,000 Google employees can take advantage of perks like free healthy and gourmet meals, laundry and fitness facilities, generous paid parental leave, and on-site childcare."
- "Employees also report that Google allows them flexibility to work on passion projects and tap into their creativity."
- "Twenty-eight percent of employees work from home or telecommute some, most, or all of the time."[24]

When I visited Google offices in Toronto, the first thing I noticed were the cafeterias on almost every floor. They offer healthy and delicious food for free, so there is no reason employees cannot enjoy nutritious breakfasts, snacks, lunches, and dinners each day. By providing this, Google is making food the center of a healthy workday. Company leaders know if they feed people healthy food, their performance is going to be better. This is directly in

24 Rachel Gillett, "5 Reasons Google Is the Best Place to Work in America and No Other Company Can Touch It," *Business Insider*, April 28, 2016, http://www.businessinsider.com/google-is-the-best-company-to-work-for-in-america-2016-4.

line with our own efforts to help employees live healthier lives through our work-life balance program. We don't want work making people sick or tired. We don't want it to drain their energy. We work to be a place that makes people healthier and better overall.

Google is also deliberate and intentional about giving employees breaks. These breaks are not about going out and having a smoke. There are beach volleyball pits, Ping-Pong tables, a music room, a meditation room, and even a small climbing wall. There are foosball tables and an area to play roller hockey. There are endless opportunities to do something active, engaging, and fun that are completely unrelated to work to allow employees to take a real break. This allows them to come back to work energized and excited.

There also are places for employees to rest. The offices have nap pods, capsules impermeable to light and sound with alarms. They are the perfect place to take a twenty-minute power nap. This shows Google cares about letting their employees recharge when they need to.

They also want to make sure their employees stimulate their minds in fun ways. There's a mobile library where they can study different languages. Employees can learn Mandarin on their lunch breaks.

Each floor also has a private cabin area where employees attend to personal affairs. If they need to make a private personal phone call or address a need at home, there's a place where they can get away from work and deal with whatever they need to. This shows while Google is intentional about separating work and family, company leaders also recognize family has a place and they support people who need to be able to tend to those matters while they're at work. This is completely in line with one of the goals of our program. One of the primary principles we've put forward is to always enable people to support their loved ones.

There is also a deliberate attempt to increase tranquility at the office. They have self-controlled massage chairs as well as on-site masseuses. They want their people to be able to take a moment, calm down, and be tranquil. They also welcome dogs at the office, which can provide both comfort and companionship to owners and contribute to an overall positive mood.

Google employees also adhere to the 80/20 rule, which dictates they spend 80 percent of their time on their primary jobs and 20 percent working on passion projects they believe will help the company. Many exciting, innovative products can trace their beginnings back to the time people have spent working on projects outside their usual job descriptions. This speaks directly to the need for companies to be creative and develop fresh solutions to stay competitive. Unless leaders enable people to take time to be intentional about being creative, they will remain stuck in the old way of working and all but guarantee their business will become irrelevant in five years.

All these components work together to help people be at their best and show how the workplace of the future can enable people to positively contribute to a company's long-term success.

AMAZON

Tech giant Amazon, the largest internet-based retailer in the world, is taking a particularly innovative approach to increasing employee happiness.

Several years ago, the company came under public scrutiny for its aggressive approach to the workplace in which employees were expected to work long hours, including weekends, be constantly reachable and, overall, be workaholics.

When designing their new $4 billion headquarters in Seattle, company leaders decided to add an unusual element to give employees a place to disconnect from work and immerse themselves in nature. They built enormous, junglelike terrariums packed with three thousand species of plants from around the world. According to the *Huff-*

ington Post article, "Amazon Is Offering a Jaw-Dropping New Perk for Its Seattle Employees," employees will have access to sixty-five thousand square feet of tropical greenery on campus. Bringing the outdoors in can have great benefits in the workplace. The article points to research from the University of Exeter, which shows office plants can increase well-being by 47 percent, creativity by 45 percent, and productivity by 38 percent.[25]

Amazon's move to bring the outdoors in is just one way company leaders can think outside of the box when deciding what will make their employees happy. Again, you may not be able to give your workplace a complete overhaul, but you don't need to. There are many ways you can create healthier work environments without being one of the Googles or Amazons of the world.

25 Alexander C. Kaufman, "Amazon Is Offering a Jaw-Dropping New Perk for Its Seattle Employees," *Huffington Post*, July 11, 2016, https://www.huffingtonpost.com/entry/amazon-seattle-domes_us_5783acc5e4b0344d51500c1c.

CHAPTER 11

The Focus Effect: Plan in Action

Work. Live. Play. These three words are used frequently in the field of real estate, when the Realtor is showing how a home can allow a person or family to do all three in an environment where they are happy and thriving. They also have a direct tie to what we are trying to do by creating a new workplace environment. Yes, we want to work. We want to work very productively, but we also want to live. Really living means you're not stressed all the time. You are healthy. You are eating well. Play is what we do with our breaks from work. A countless number of studies show stress is one of the leading causes of almost all illness. We need a world where we do more than just work and die.

We've created a step-by-step protocol to follow to make sure this doesn't happen.

The changes proposed in this book are meant to be introduced and implemented gradually in stages. When launching our own program, we found people appreciated the slow implementation of it. Had we given them everything at once, they would have become discouraged and the changes wouldn't last.

The following is a twelve-week plan we've designed for leaders to follow when putting the program into place in their own companies.

WEEK 1: START WITH "WHY?"

The first step you must take before even starting the program is making sure everybody is on board with it. Have the representatives who are running the program present it to management first, and make sure they understand exactly what the program and its goals are. Educate the board so all members know what's happening. Get all higher-ups prepared for the change so there is company-wide understanding of what's coming.

Then a huge component of implementation is educating the employees about what the program is and is not. They must understand this is not about trying to find a way to squeeze more out of them. This is about having an educational discussion about how we got to this point of incessant distraction as a society, the impact it is having on our well-being and productivity, and steps we can all take together to improve. Leadership must be willing to admit it has unintentionally contributed to the problem by allowing 24/7 access to employees. This is a good time to tell them what you will do in your role in helping them reclaim their evenings and weekends. As an employer, you want to convey the message that they are entitled to their time off. Again, you can do this with newsletters, lunch-and-learn sessions, or other creative methods.

In the early days, people might express concerns that stem back to a lack of understanding. They might fear reducing the time they work will be frowned on. They might assume if they prove they can get the same amount of work done in five hours, another supervisor will give them three or four more hours of work.

1% TIP: SHARE THE VISION

At the beginning of the twelve-week process of creating a culture of focus, take ample time to ensure that everyone understands the vision: a healthier, more productive, more balanced workplace that is both more successful and more enjoyable.

Everyone must understand that fewer work hours does not mean anyone is going to be punished in any way or made to feel bad because of how they've been working to this point. Employees should still expect to be paid as much as they were for working more hours. It's about productivity. If I can get the same or greater productivity from an employee in six hours than I was getting before in nine hours, why wouldn't I be happy with that as an employer? Management must convey that they are simply trying to right the ship with the intention of making employees happier, healthier, and more inclined to stay with the company longer.

They must understand we're not trying to squeeze more blood out of the stone. We're saying the stone's not working well. Employees are getting sick, burned out, overweight, and stressed because of the way they are living and working outside and inside the workplace. By introducing this new way of working, we can change all of that and create more productive, efficient employees.

The single most important thing to start with is a shared, clear vision of the future. There's a reason Simon Sinek's book, *Start with Why*, is so popular. There is great value in identifying motivations behind actions and helping everyone to see the bigger picture. When you take time to figure out the why, you are better equipped to overcome any challenges to the new way of doing things that might arise in your life or workplace. Tell employees why you are doing this. If you're clear about why you are going to do this, everyone will feel more motivated to get on board.

WEEK 2: DECONSTRUCTION

At this point, it's time to deconstruct what you're currently doing and build a better plan. By deconstruction we mean taking a step back and examining what you're currently doing. How are you spending your time? Where is your focus? Break that down to smaller parts so you can rebuild a better workday. It's a way of constantly rebuilding yourself so you can constantly be better, stronger, faster, and more efficient. A great example of the importance of deconstruction was the philosophy of elBulli, a Michelin three-star restaurant in Spain (now closed), which was open for a limited season each year. For six months of the year, it would close to source new ingredients, develop menu items, and come up with new systems and processes.

Week 2 is when both leadership and staff do a current state of the union. Ask one another, how much is everyone working? What are the current hours that everybody's currently putting in? What's the current effectiveness? How productive is the group? What are the stress levels of the group? What's the health of the group? What's the performance of the group? What business metrics can you track to determine if the change is effective?

Deconstruct as much as possible within the organization to determine where you are starting. This will later help you measure the effectiveness of the program. If you don't get a clear metric outlined at the beginning of the project, you cannot track your progress to determine whether improvements are being made. Quite often, we make dramatic improvements but forget to take a moment to look back at how far we've come. It's hard to do that unless you have baseline data to assess.

As previously mentioned, it can help to have employees track email time before and after changes are implemented so they can see the dramatic difference more focused work time can make. It can also help to look at how many files the accounting staff can tend to each day before and after.

Also measure sick days. Look at how many days employees missed for the last three years before the program was implemented and compare the data with how many days are missed for six months after. In all likelihood, you will see a significant reduction in sick days and benefit costs.

Measure employee satisfaction. In our pilot, many employees kept personal journals detailing their weight loss, improved sleep, and general sense of feeling better and more engaged.

Do a benefits analysis. How much are employees spending on drugs and health care? From a leadership perspective, look at how you are doing as far as recruitment and retention. Any way you can measure what people are doing before and after beginning the program will help you see how performance can increase in an environment with fewer distractions.

There are several ways you can gather this information. You can take a poll or create a Google form for people to fill out. You can have staff meetings or one-on-one meetings. Regardless of how you go about it, at the end, you should have clear understanding of where you are as a company and what needs to happen to move you forward.

WEEK 3: SEPARATE WORK AND HOME

This week is about shifting from working all the time and trying to catch up on home tasks while we are at work to creating boundaries between the two. Now employees should understand when they are at work, they are expected to be fully at work. When they are at home, they are fully at home. If they are working from home, there is a defined time they work before engaging with their families. As more employers offer work-from-home options for employees, it is key a proper structure is in place that allows people to work uninterrupted and understand the clear distinction between work time and downtime.

Email policies, such as those outlined in chapter 6, should be in place. Pick a day and communicate that from that point on, employees will not receive or respond to emails outside of work hours. Have employees set up autoresponders, or even better, have the IT department set the servers so they don't send or receive emails during those hours. Senders can get a bounce back explaining the policy and offering a link where they can reach someone if the matter is urgent.

Employees should also understand there will be times throughout the day when they are expected to go without their phones. Expect a little bit of initial panic at this. They will say, "What if my children or my spouse or the teachers need to get hold of me?" That's a level of anxiety most people have. In reality, most people seldom have even one catastrophic emergency a year, and the likelihood of it occurring during work hours is slim. Statistically, it's not near as real as the ever-present anxiety about it would suggest. But to soothe any concerns, provide a number, perhaps one assigned to a secretary or assistant, that friends and family can call in the event of an emergency. When we implemented our program, this is the area where we received the most initial pushback. People were concerned their families would not be able to reach them when they really needed them. Reassure them by creating dedicated lines to field such calls, and remind them they can always connect with loved ones during breaks and lunches.

Feeling like you always have to check your phone contributes to feelings of exhaustion and burnout. Not long ago, most parents never felt the need to check in with their children multiple times throughout the day, whereas now, it's almost uncommon for elementary-age children to not have cell phones. No one is doing anyone any good by reinforcing the idea that that level of connectivity and anxiety is acceptable. As parents, we've created an environment where kids feel like they always have to be accessible to us. We need to understand the impact it has on children when we expect them to be constantly connected to us. They see it as normal and will expect it from others as well, thus perpetuating the idea that we can never be out of reach.

You will have introduced the concept of single-tasking,

and by decreasing the amount of time they are spending jumping back and forth between work and home tasks, this should come easily.

WEEK 4: EAT SMARTER

Employers must be able to give their people the tools, tactics, and strategies they need to focus better and have more energy. One of the easiest ways to do that is to help people eat smarter.

By week 4, you should be encouraging people to deliberately begin to create new habits and routines around healthy eating. The company can start providing healthy snacks and drinks and eliminating unhealthy options. It's time to get rid of the high-calorie, low-nutrient offerings such as pop, juice, and vending machine junk. It's time to start investing in good coffee, healthy water, herbal tea, and healthy snacks.

Consider catering healthy lunches or identifying places nearby where people can go to get a healthy lunch. Look to decrease the amount of simple carbohydrates such as rice, bread, and pasta, and move people toward vegetables, fruits, and healthy protein sources.

We also want to get people considering using healthy fats during the day such as avocado, olive oil, coconut, and wild fish. These foods elevate omega-3 fatty acid levels and make an enormous difference in brain power over time. This is, after all, about giving people more energy. They will avoid the afternoon crash, which is usually caused by the foods they eat at lunch, and provide people with the snacks they need to be able to sustain their energy all day.

If you eliminate the "bad" snacks, particularly from vending machines, you might be met with an uproar initially. I recommend a graduated implementation where you slowly replace unhealthy options with healthy options. The reality is, if the unhealthy stuff is there, people are going to eat it. Your environment largely dictates your success.

1% TIP: CHANGE PEOPLE'S THINKING ABOUT FOOD

There are enormous benefits to small changes in the way we eat. Working to shift the food culture of your organization will create a context that will improve the health and wellness of your employees and enable them to be more effective and successful. We are all highly influenced by what goes on around us, so companies have an opportunity to shift the way their teams function through simple things such as a shift in thinking about food.

Google has a very interesting system when it comes to food. Foods in the cafeteria are labeled green, yellow, and red. The green foods are the things you can eat as much as you want: vegetables, fruits, and healthy proteins and fats.

Yellow foods—slightly higher calorie, lower-nutrient-type foods—should be eaten only every once in a while. The red foods are the desserts: high-sugar, crisis-time food. It is very clear what is good for you and what is not. What you do depends on your company's culture.

Remember, this doesn't have to be expensive. The costs can be shared with employees if need be. We found many healthy options from local vendors for less than six dollars when implementing our program. We covered the entire cost, but even if it needs to be shared, the benefits to all parties are well worth the money spent.

Nutrition can be very confusing and controversial, but if you break it down, it's all very simple. You just need to take in as much nutrition as you can in as few calories as possible. Easy changes such as avoiding processed foods and eating more fresh fruits and vegetables can make a world of difference. Look to decrease your intake of sugar and highly processed carbs. Add proteins in the morning to help you concentrate and healthy fats to improve brain function. Keep everything as simple as possible by following a few rules, and you can dramatically improve your health and work performance.

WEEK 5: ELIMINATE DISTRACTIONS

This is the week when you will ask people to deliberately

start eliminating distractions and working within a tight level of total focus. People should designate a time when they will be completely focused on one task.

In chapter 4, we asked you to think critically about when you do your best work and then build a daily routine around that. Now you must ask your employees to do the same.

Humans all have circadian rhythms. We're naturally responsive to a light-dark cycle that occurs with the sun and the moon. Every human has certain times during the day when they are going to be more alert and able to concentrate better. The peak performance window for a lot of people is typically about three to four hours during the day, and that varies for each person.

Ask people to think about when during the day they naturally and easily do their best work, and encourage them to work those hours. Remember, for some, that might mean working outside the normal nine-to-five. Some people excel in the mornings; some people are more nocturnal. As long as it does not interfere with the day-to-day function and productivity of the company, employees should be able to work when they work best.

Working at your ideal time while devoid of distraction sets the stage for entering flow, that time and space when we have plenty of energy, we're focused, we're excited, we're engaged, work is easy, and time becomes irrelevant. Everyone has probably felt that at one time in their life that natural getting into the zone, getting into the flow. Lead performers can enter flow on demand by controlling their arousal state. If you're not motivated, bored, tired, nervous, stressed, anxious, or fearful, you cannot perform. If you're motivated, focused, and dialed in, you can get great work done.

1% TIP: HELP YOUR STAFF UNDERSTAND THEIR OWN RHYTHMS

Leading your team through a process of understanding their own circadian rhythm is a simple and powerful basis for helping them work more efficiently. When they understand the times that they are most productive, they can then implement systems to protect that time and optimize the value of time at work and in their personal lives, which will elevate the overall value of everything the organization does.

As an employer, you can take advantage of employees' preferred work times. For example, if one is an early bird and the other likes the afternoon, they can basically cover each other in the overlap. This shows how you can reduce hours within certain departments that have that ability to cross-train.

Once people know when they will work, they must commit to staying on task. They should turn off:

- all computer notifications
- email
- social media alerts
- phone ringers

They can close their doors, if possible, or put a sign up that says, "Deep focused. Please help me concentrate." They can do whatever it takes to completely shut out distractions so they can focus on single tasks during their devoted work time.

WEEK 6: EMAIL BATCHING

The frequency with which we check email is the biggest interruption we all face at work. We feel like we must keep checking email so we stay on top of it. To deal with that, I recommend email batching, which is doing emails at very specific times during the day. If you need a refresher on batching, refer to chapter 8.

When encouraging employees to batch email, you must educate them on how it works. Say, "If you're able to respond to one hundred emails in one hour, let's break that into three pockets during the course of the day. For example, if you start your workday at 9:00 a.m. and we determine you need three stops during the day to do emails, maybe you work from 9:00 a.m. to 9:50 a.m. on task. Then, from 9:50 a.m. until 10:10 a.m., you spend twenty minutes cleaning up your emails. When you're doing that, you're not doing anything else. When you're done, you will not check email again until 1:30 p.m."

Now the employee understands he is not expected to be constantly looking for emails. He can look at his email flow during the day and ask himself, "How often do I need to check them? How long on average does it take me to respond to them?" Then he can build those times into his day so he is no longer dealing with them nonstop.

WEEK 7: THE WORK-REST PRINCIPLE

The work-rest principle is a practice whereby you alternate periods of focused intense work with periods of deliberate rest, recovery, and regeneration. An example would be Tony Schwartz's 90-Minute Solution from The Energy Project, in which people work in ninety-minute increments followed by thirty-minute breaks. Our colleague Robin Sharma advocates sixty-minute work blocks followed by a ten-minute break. You can create whatever timetable works best for you, but we recommend a maximum work interval should be ninety minutes or less with minimum rest period of ten minutes.

The goal is to create a situation where someone knows that they've got a stretch of time when they can really focus, be as undistracted as possible, be hyperproductive, but then take a break to recover and regenerate. Now, instead of operating constantly at 80 percent, people can work at 100 percent and then commit 100 percent to their thirty-minute recovery and regeneration period. The result is improved performance and better health, as breaks are key to eliminating symptoms of chronic stress and anxiety.

> ### 1% TIP: RESPECT RECOVERY AND REST
>
> It is often the norm in a corporate setting for downtime to be viewed as slacking off or a lack of a work ethic. You can help to change that by assisting everyone in understanding the role that deliberate downtime plays in amplifying the productivity of work.

The important thing is to incorporate regular breaks into your workday. This is likely a new concept for many people who, for most of their careers, have been cramming in as much work to as many hours as they can, day in and day out. Allowing for periods of rest within your day will move you toward a different way of working, the aforementioned Power Work. This can mean working for sixty minutes with fifteen off, working for ninety minutes with thirty off, or whatever works for you. The key is to find a cadence that allows you to up your game, improve the quality of your work, and improve your physical and mental health. And when you take breaks, really take a break—go for a walk, get away from the office, step away from work completely.

WEEK 8: SINGLE-TASKING

As discussed in chapter 2, humans are incapable of multitasking. It's physiologically impossible. Our brains work best when we focus on one thing at a time.

According to the *Harvard Business Review*,[26] "focused managers aren't in reactive mode; they choose not to respond immediately to every issue that comes their way or get sidetracked from their goals by distractions like email, meetings, setbacks, and unforeseen demands. Because they have a clear understanding of what they want to accomplish, they carefully weigh their options before selecting a course of action. Moreover, because they commit to only one or two key projects, they can devote their full attention to the projects they believe in."

To improve your own mental focus, try single-tasking.

---

26 Heike Bruch and Sumantra Ghoshal, "Beware the Busy Manager," *Harvard Business Review*, February 2002, https://hbr.org/2002/02/beware-the-busy-manager.

Single-tasking demands we pick the most important task to work on first and perform that task as exclusively as possible until it is either complete or we are out of whatever time we allotted for the job.

Week 8 is the time to ask people to build the opportunity to single-task on the most important things they need to get done. Once they do, they will see amazing efficiencies emerge and be able to do splendid work with less effort.

1% TIP: CELEBRATE SINGLE-TASKING

There are some deeply held beliefs about the value of doing many things at once. By helping your teams understand the energy and efficiency loss associated with managing several things at the same time, you can help them dramatically improve their efficiency and well-being.

You can encourage them to set timers so they are not always looking at the clock. If they work on multiple screens, suggest they cut back to one, provided it doesn't interfere with their responsibilities.

Management must present single-tasking as something simple for people to do. They can start by identifying one hour of every single day when they can work with no distractions. If that is successful, ask them to find a second hour block. In time, the practice will become routine.

Some tips for single-tasking include:

- Organizing your tasks before you start the day. Set aside specific times to focus solely on the high-priority activities.
- Batching emails and phone calls
- Working off one screen
- Turning off notifications
- Meditating for a few minutes before starting focused time of work
- Putting measures in place to stave off any anticipated interruptions
- Scheduling walks or other rewards throughout the day

If we focus, we can do more in less time, which makes better use of our energy. Try it and see how it works for you.

WEEK 9: PRIORITY MANAGEMENT

One of the things I found to be unbelievably helpful with the employees I've been working with is shifting from time management to priority management. Time management is living by your calendar. Priority management is getting the most important things you need to do every day done.

We need to identify the most important things we need to do in our lives, be they personal, professional, health-related, or work-related, and schedule them during the times of the day when we have the most energy. Don't just schedule meetings—schedule everything important to you. Schedule workouts. Schedule a monthly dinner out with your spouse. Schedule playtime with your kids. Do it so those activities don't get lost. Let your priorities dictate how you live your life. As you live your day, so you live your life. If you are scheduling the urgent things and never getting to the important things, that's a recipe for short-term frustration and long-term unhappiness.

If you don't make working out or spending time with your loved ones as important as your next meeting, they won't happen. You have to learn to make sure workouts and downtime are part of your schedule. Even if you are traveling, set aside time to meet with a trainer or just take a long walk.

1% TIP: DO WHAT MATTERS THE MOST

Corporations are infamous for bogging down in a range of urgent or seemingly important issues that aren't actually adding value. By helping your teams shift from time management (living by the calendar) to priority management (doing the most important things well), you can create a wave of focus and wellness.

You must make sure your activities are consistent with your dreams, goals, and objectives. You want your actions to map to your ambitions. A lot of people get busy and end up losing months just being busy and not getting anything real done. One way you can better manage your priorities is to list all of your roles and responsibilities and rank them from most to least important. Then make sure that on a daily basis, you are allocating specific time during the time of day when your energy levels are highest to work on your highest priority tasks in a completely undistracted manner. If you can do this consistently over a period, you will make tremendous progress toward achieving your dreams. Also, be prepared to defend your dedicated on-task time. Do not be afraid to communicate your commitment to your priorities to the people around you and keep these decisions in mind as you go about your daily life. Evaluate your objectives constantly so you can construct your ideal day, week, month, year, and life.

To do this, you might have to break away from the belief that you have to respond to every email, voice mail, text message, and so forth, on the same day you receive it. I used to fall into this trap, thinking it was rude to do otherwise. Some messages can go unanswered; others should be blocked entirely. If you are spending too much time fielding unsolicited messages, block, unsubscribe, or delete—do whatever you have to do to keep such distractions from stealing your time.

WEEK 10: MIND AND BODY CONNECTION—BODY

This week is about educating employees on the link between the body and the mind and how we can supercharge the brain by moving our bodies. The only way to get your brain functioning at its absolute best is by making sure you're physically active.

You don't need to go to the gym for an hour every day—although if you do, that's great. Walking for just five minutes improves brain function. Taking the stairs or stretching does as well. We just need to sprinkle physical activity throughout the day, and if you can do that, you're going to experience many positive benefits. We know that if you can work out more intensely, the benefits increase.

Treat this week as a call to action to get people to understand if they add physical activity to their days, the time investment will come back to them exponentially in returns.

Encourage them to book it in their calendars and make it as important as their most important business meeting, because it is. If someone wants to schedule something with you at the same time, don't allow it, just as you would not cancel an important meeting. And employers, don't make employees feel guilty for taking the time to take a walk or get in a quick workout during the day. You should be encouraging such behavior, not making people think they'll be punished for doing it.

At home, you can carve out time to walk with loved ones, play ball, or go to the park. Consider blocking out TV for certain hours. It's too easy to come home, turn on the TV, and lose endless hours to sitting in front of it. Perhaps even try TV fasting for a week or two. At the end, consider how much more free time you had and what you were able to do with it.

Finally, if you feel your body beginning to experience the effects of stress, STOP: Stop, Take a breath, Observe, and Proceed. Stop whatever you are doing and become aware of the present moment. Take a breath (or two or ten) very slowly, a few seconds in, a few out. Observe your body and scan it for any tensions you can work to release. Then proceed, or carry on with your life. Set an intention guided by what's most important and move forward. This kind of mindfulness can be very powerful in bringing you into the present moment and raising your awareness, allowing you to perform at a higher level with greater focus.

WEEK 11: MIND AND BODY CONNECTION—MIND

Mindfulness can be just as important as physical activity. Even five minutes a day spent controlling your attention and allowing your mind to relax has incredible benefits. It can lower stress, anxiety, depression, and incidence of chronic disease; it can also increase focus and concentration. It is one of the most powerful things humans can do to improve mental health and performance.

Many of the leaders who are revolutionizing the business world right now practice some form of meditation. There are many resources available for those looking to introduce meditation into their daily lives. I recommend Headspace.com, Calm.com (both also available as smartphone apps), the Muse headband, or the Breathe app on Apple Watch.

By introducing this concept to employees, you can again expect them to decrease their workday by another thirty minutes. By practicing mindfulness, one's ability to control his attention the rest of the day improves dramatically. He is distracted less and able to focus more deeply. A little bit of training results in an exponential return in terms of productivity. There are also many health benefits to mindfulness, including lower levels of stress and lower blood pressure.

WEEK 12: LIFE ENGINEERING/PURSUING DREAMS

The last step is all about consolidating gains, celebrating progress, and assessing how far you've come. This is the time to revisit the initial assessment you conducted during the deconstruction phase. Ask the same questions and measure your gains. Make this process fun by planning a lunch around it, handing out awards for significant improvements, or incorporating some fun challenges and contests.

Once they see how much "extra" time they now have, employees should be encouraged to be deliberate about doing something with it. If they have gone through the program well, they should end up with three hours a day they didn't have before. Humans are very good at replacing things. Unless they fill the time with something else, it's likely they will simply go back to working again.

> ### 1% TIP: INDIVIDUAL DREAMS
> ### AND COLLECTIVE SUCCESS
>
> When people go after their dreams, they are energized, focused, and passionate about their work. Organizations that make it a priority to understand what people want out of their work and life create a culture that buzzes with excitement and possibility.

Challenge people to find things to do that will move them forward in life. Ask them, "Can you take a course? Do you want to spend more time with your family? Will you start working out more? Maybe it's time to begin massage therapy. Maybe you want to be out in nature." Encourage them to do things they enjoy tremendously that also better their lives. This "life engineering" helps us figure out how we can do things differently and spend our time doing the things we absolutely love to do.

Now is the time to reap the reward of the changes you all have implemented. The company wants employees to reward themselves by allowing them to have lives. Do an employee satisfaction survey to see the significant difference in how people feel. Don't be surprised if everyone is much happier and healthier.

COACHING AND ACCOUNTABILITY

Coaching and accountability are two things you will have to pay special attention to throughout the implementation of the program. You will have to check in with your people regularly to make sure they are doing what's expected, as well as gauging their feelings toward to the changes. You might even appoint someone to be in charge of this.

One-on-one meetings can come in handy. We conducted them at the beginning, midway through, and with exit interviews. In between meetings, it helps if the person at the company overseeing the implementation is visible and accessible to employees for even casual conversations related to the changes. They can hang out in the lunchroom and simply ask, "How's everything going? What's working for you? What isn't? Why?" If it is a week when a new strategy is introduced, ask if they've tried it. If they say no, offer them more details and encourage them to give it a shot. These encounters can prove just as fruitful as anything more formal.

They also provide coaching opportunities if the employees

have any questions. You cannot implement changes if you feel like you are acting on your own. You really do need someone to work with who can help guide you.

While company leaders can help, it can also be beneficial to have a designated accountability partner. If you work together with a colleague or coworker to implement these changes together, and you talk about it and hold each other accountable for actually doing it, the results can be amazing. Encourage employees to find someone else in the organization to check in with regularly and discuss their experiences with the changes.

Another option is creating teams. Typically, around six to eight people is the perfect team size. These people will work together to implement the principles systematically and consistently. They all do the same thing at the same time progressively throughout the program, and in doing so, the likelihood of it being successful long term is exponentially greater.

Life Mastery Checklist

OVERVIEW

Living your best life is an exercise in mastering your personal life and your work. These two components influence each other greatly, and some of the most successful companies in the world are also the ones that have been most innovative in promoting work-life balance and creating work environments that enable people to be their best. For example, Google and Amazon have a unique approach to workplace culture that has been proven to foster creativity, wellness, and a huge return on investment of capital and time. These companies are a model for how organizations can support employees in achieving life mastery.

THE QUIZ

Answer the questions below to assess the culture of your

organization related to focus, wellness, and productivity. Your responses will assist you in identifying simple changes you can make to get more out of your time, enjoy your life and work, and elevate your performance individually and as a group.

DIRECTIONS

Select the answer that best matches your current situation. Your responses will give you a sense of how you are supporting your ability to achieve the Focus Effect. Add up your scores at the end to see how you're doing. You can then make minor changes by addressing one question at a time. Then come back in a couple of months to take the quiz again and see how your focus has improved!

1. DO YOU SHARE YOUR VISION FOR A CULTURE OF FOCUS?

- Always (5 points)
- Yup (4 points)
- Pretty much (3 points)
- Sort of (2 points)
- Not really (1 point)
- Never (0 points)

Recommendations: Take ample time to ensure that everyone understands the organizational vision of the cultural change you are trying to enable: a healthier, more productive, more balanced workplace that is both more successful and more enjoyable.

Rationale: Change is very difficult for people under normal circumstances and even more of a challenge when you ask them to alter some of their basic conceptions of how they work. Letting them all in on the vision up front and taking the time to make sure they understand how improved focus can benefit them and the organization will go a long way toward their ability to participate wholeheartedly. Ultimately, change is most effective when individuals and groups are empowered to come up with creative solutions that achieve the vision, but that means they have to understand why it is a priority and how it will benefit them.

2. CAN YOU DECONSTRUCT YOUR CURRENT APPROACH TO WORK?

- Always (5 points)
- Yup (4 points)
- Pretty much (3 points)
- Sort of (2 points)
- Not really (1 point)
- Never (0 points)

Recommendations: Audit distractions, inefficiencies, and stressors across the entire organization to build a better plan. Do this by taking a step back, examining everything, and breaking it down into smaller parts. How are you spending your time? Where is your focus? How much is everyone working? What are the current hours that everybody's currently putting in? What's the current effectiveness? How productive is the group? What are the stress levels of the group? What's the health of the group? What's the performance of the group? What business metrics can you track to determine if the change is effective?

Rationale: The only way to constantly rebuild the organization and ensure that you can continually be better, stronger, faster, and more efficient is to commit to understanding what is happening now and see how it might improve.

3. DO YOU SEPARATE WORK AND HOME?

- Always (5 points)
- Yup (4 points)
- Pretty much (3 points)
- Sort of (2 points)
- Not really (1 point)
- Never (0 points)

Recommendations: Implement personal practices and corporate policies that create a clear line between work time and home time.

Rationale: By amplifying the quality of work and protecting the need for genuine recovery and rest away from the job, you can dramatically improve the well-being of employees and the success of the company. You can also eliminate the creep of personal concerns becoming a major distraction during the workday. With creative solutions such as a company policy that limits time for email, you can create a culture not just of focus but of excellence.

4. DO YOU CREATE A CULTURE OF HEALTHY FOOD?

- Always (5 points)
- Yup (4 points)
- Pretty much (3 points)
- Sort of (2 points)
- Not really (1 point)
- Never (0 points)

Recommendations: Make an organization-wide commitment to supporting employees in a shift to healthy food options. Change what's in the vending machine. Change the food in the cafeteria. Change what is ordered in for meetings and parties. And take time to provide everyone with ample education about Power Fuel and how it impacts them.

Rationale: Changing the way we eat is one of the biggest personal challenges for just about anyone who tries. These changes are much easier if the entire organization is set up to support healthy food choices that lead to productive, enjoyable, and energized living and working. Everyone is better positioned to change their approach to nutrition if they are supported by the community around them.

5. DO YOU ELIMINATE DISTRACTIONS?

- Always (5 points)
- Yup (4 points)
- Pretty much (3 points)
- Sort of (2 points)
- Not really (1 point)
- Never (0 points)

Recommendations: Make a detailed assessment of the diverse range of distractions that detract from productive work and then commit to eliminating them, individually and collectively. Change your attitude to notifications, interruptions, multitasking, socializing during the workday, and managing personal affairs while at work. Help everyone establish an attitude that when you work, you work, and when you play, you play.

Rationale: We can all control the impact of distractions in our lives, and if the organization makes a commitment to doing so, a cultural shift is possible.

6. DO YOU MAKE EMAIL BATCHING THE NORM?

- Always (5 points)
- Yup (4 points)
- Pretty much (3 points)
- Sort of (2 points)
- Not really (1 point)
- Never (0 points)

Recommendations: Establish a culture around email that empowers people to manage their email at particular times of the day and not check it when they are engaged in other tasks.

Rationale: Email is one of the most invasive distractions that can undermine a culture of focus, and organizations need to be proactive about dealing with the detrimental effect that constant communication demands have on everyone. When people know that it is a supported practice to check emails at particular times and that it is OK not to be on email when they are at home, there will be a widespread sense of relief and an improvement in wellness and productivity because people will work more effectively and recover more fully when they are at home.

7. DO YOU APPLY THE WORK-REST PRINCIPLE?

- Always (5 points)
- Yup (4 points)

- Pretty much (3 points)
- Sort of (2 points)
- Not really (1 point)
- Never (0 points)

Recommendations: The work-rest principle is a practice whereby you alternate periods of focused intense work with periods of deliberate rest, recovery, and regeneration. Rather than trying to work all day long and operating at 80 percent efficiency, it's better to work at close to 100 percent for a focused period, usually ninety minutes, and then leave the workspace to spend roughly thirty minutes taking an active break.

Rationale: The human brain can focus for only ninety minutes at a time before it needs a substantial break to restore blood glucose and oxygen. Grinding it out for longer than that is unrealistic and will slowly erode quality of work and overall well-being.

8. DO YOU ENCOURAGE SINGLE-TASKING?

- Always (5 points)
- Yup (4 points)
- Pretty much (3 points)
- Sort of (2 points)
- Not really (1 point)
- Never (0 points)

Recommendations: Single-tasking demands we pick the most important task to work on first and perform that task as exclusively as possible until it is either complete or we are out of whatever time we allotted for the job. We can use this approach by being deliberate, including the following techniques: organize your tasks before you start the day with specific times for high-priority activities, batch emails and phone calls, work off one screen, turn off notifications, meditate for a few minutes before starting focused work, stave off anticipated interruptions, and schedule walks and other rewards throughout the day.

Rationale: Humans are incapable of multitasking. It's physiologically impossible. Our brains work best when we focus on one thing at a time. Ask people to single-task the most important things they need to get done, and you will see amazing efficiencies emerge that lead to splendid work with less effort.

9. DO YOU MANAGE PRIORITIES, NOT TIME?

- Always (5 points)
- Yup (4 points)
- Pretty much (3 points)
- Sort of (2 points)
- Not really (1 point)
- Never (0 points)

Recommendations: Time management is living by your calendar. Priority management is doing the most important things you need to do every day. By shifting the focus of your planning, individuals and organizations can commit time to what matters, rather than just being more efficient at whatever is currently on the agenda. One way for a person to better manage priorities is to list all of their roles and responsibilities and rank them from most to least important. Then they can ensure that they are allocating energy to the most important roles on a daily basis.

Rationale: The world around us will always make demands on our time, but we get to decide how we respond. Making an effort to live focused on your priorities will lead you to your ideal life.

10. DO YOU USE PHYSICAL ACTIVITY TO FUEL OPTIMAL PERFORMANCE?

- Always (5 points)
- Yup (4 points)
- Pretty much (3 points)
- Sort of (2 points)
- Not really (1 point)
- Never (0 points)

Recommendations: The only way to get your brain

functioning at its absolute best is by making sure you're physically active. You don't need to go to the gym for an hour everyday—although if you do, that's great. Walking for just five minutes improves brain function. Taking the stairs or stretching does as well. You just need to sprinkle physical activity throughout the day, and if you can do that, you're going to experience many positive benefits that increase as you increase the intensity of the activity. Organizations that make physical activity part of their culture encourage employees to excel in all areas of their work and lives.

Rationale: Research is unequivocal about this: The more active you are, the more supercharged you will be. Exercise improves everything from creativity to energy levels, mood, and problem solving.

11. DO YOU PRACTICE MINDFULNESS?

- Always (5 points)
- Yup (4 points)
- Pretty much (3 points)
- Sort of (2 points)
- Not really (1 point)
- Never (0 points)

Recommendations: When an organization makes a commitment to mindfulness practice, these activities begin to become normal for everyone. In whatever manner makes sense for them, introduce some form of mindfulness or meditation into employees' work lives. It can begin with just five minutes a day to clear the mind by focusing on breathing. Then it can grow to the use of mindfulness resources such as Headspace.com, Calm.com (both also available as smartphone apps), the Muse headband, or the Breathe app on the Apple Watch. There are also hundreds of courses and online resources for meditation and mindfulness.

Rationale: Increasing mindfulness is one of the most powerful things humans can do to improve mental health and performance. It can be just as important as physical activity. Even five minutes a day spent controlling your attention and allowing your mind to relax has incredible benefits. It can lower stress, anxiety, depression, and incidence of chronic disease; it can also increase focus and concentration. There are other health benefits as well, including lower levels of stress and lower blood pressure.

12. DO YOU SET SOME DREAMS?

- Always (5 points)
- Yup (4 points)
- Pretty much (3 points)
- Sort of (2 points)
- Not really (1 point)
- Never (0 points)

Recommendations: Dream setting is about expressing what you most want to accomplish in your life and making a plan to go after it. It's about thinking big, reaching high, and tapping into your greatest passions. When people commit themselves to deliberately pursuing dreams, their lives and work are imbued with energy and focus.

Rationale: Life is what we make of it. By expressing and committing to our dreams, we can all make them happen. It's just a matter of knowing what you really want to achieve and going after it.

TOTAL SCORE

40+ points:
You are living the dream! You have set up your life to optimize your focus and ensure you perform at your best most of the time.

20–39 points:
You are getting there. Keep tweaking your approach to find more areas for focus in your life.

0–19 points:
You have made a start but there is work to be done. Pick one item from the quiz above and work on it this week. After you have made some changes in that area, you can come back and focus on another area for improvement.

PART 4

Global Implications

. . . .

*If you love what you do and are willing to do what
it takes, it's within your reach.*

—STEVE WOZNIAK

CHAPTER 12

A Call to Action

We don't want this to be just another book about how to work differently. We want to address the global issue of unhealthy attachment to distraction we are experiencing, how that's affecting the human race, and how it's also significantly impacting the workplace. This issue needs to be seen in the big picture.

We are moving from an industrial-based economy to a technology-based economy, and as a result, there is massive disruption that's only going to get more intense. We are only twenty years into the internet. We are just getting started. As a result, being married to the traditional ways of doing things is no longer feasible. We need to map out a way of working that is going to enable us to do things differently in the future and to enable workers and companies of the future to respond to the fact that many tasks are going to be automated. We need to enable people to be creative and more agile with their thinking. The only way to do that is by adopting the types of strategies we are proposing in this book and program.

Although we are speaking about a new way of working, it's really about setting the stage for the future and putting people in a position where they can respond instead of reacting. This is a critical foundation for us to consider before we move forward.

People often lose sight of the fact that most employers do care about the best interests of their employees. Everybody wants what's best for everybody else so we can all lead our happiest, best lives. The problem is that either they haven't been able to identify the issues and/or they don't have the solutions.

We didn't even notice when it became OK for people to talk and text through meetings. There was no one day when it suddenly became acceptable to email employees during dinner. It just crept in. But we allowed it to creep in, and now we must deal with it. There are many good employers who do want better for their employees but just don't know how to undo what's been done.

Yet if we do nothing, we continue to contribute to the biggest health threats to the human race today. Obesity and poor mental health statistics are staggering and continue to climb. The number of people who are sleep deprived is constantly on the rise. It is time to reclaim our health, both physical and mental.

WORDS OF WISDOM: CHAD REMPEL

Professional football player Chad Rempel is a Grey Cup champion with the Canadian Football League. As a long snapper, he relies on focus and eliminating distractions to do his very specialized job. In his early days, he would practice by doing a thousand reps each night.

"The performer who focuses the best wins the most," he says.

After winning the Grey Cup in 2012, he decided to master the skill and focus on only long snapping. His efforts paid off and landed him a spot on the Chicago Bears in the NFL. It was not about volume anymore; every single rep was a championship kick. Anything could happen in the game, and nothing would affect him.

"If your mind wanders at all, you cannot do a good snap," he says.

Rempel has one thought before taking the field: "Finish the snap," which he eventually refined down into just "Finish." A single word is all it takes for him to focus.

At thirty-one years old, he was the oldest drafted player ever signed to the Chicago Bears. Everyone doubted him. No one believed he could make the move from the CFL to the NFL. He blocked all that noise out and worked consistently on mastery.

"Do good work and good things will happen," he says. "I'm constantly in the pursuit of perfection."

This is not a problem that's going to solve itself. All of

us—employees and employers—have created it, whether passively or actively, and it's up to all of us to fix it. We must stay competitive in a world where artificial intelligence threatens to render us irrelevant. Many fields of industry are already affected—medicine, driving, law, customer service—and soon, countless others will be as well. We must adapt to survive, and we cannot do that with an outdated, obsolete way of working and living.

Start by creating an evolution in your own personal life, then apply what you've learned and experienced to your workplace. Remember, as you live your day, so you live your life. Even if you start with just finding fifteen more minutes in a day, you are moving in the right direction. You will begin to reclaim control over your life and stop distractions from stealing your time.

We encourage you, as you continue on your journey, to engage in the community. Follow us on social media and at www.thefocuseffect.ca.

In doing so, you will contribute to a future where all people have the chance to reach their potential and live their best lives.

About the Authors

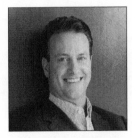

DR. GREG WELLS is an assistant professor of kinesiology at the University of Toronto, associate scientist of physiology and experimental medicine at The Hospital for Sick Children, and former director of sport science at the Canadian Sport Institute. He served as analyst for CTV for two Olympic Games, has coached dozens of elite athletes, and has competed in numerous tests of athleticism, including Ironman Canada. He is author of *Superbodies: Peak Performance Secrets from the World's Best Athletes* and *The Ripple Effect*.

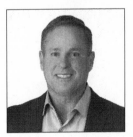

BRUCE BOWSER, president and CEO of AMJ Campbell Van Lines, is known for his ability to create high-performance workplace cultures that produce results. He has grown his company from $34 million at his appointment to president in 1997 to more than $200 million today. He also has held management positions with the Bank of Nova Scotia. He is a licensed pilot and avid golfer and hockey player.

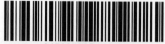

Made in the USA
Columbia, SC
02 May 2018